Media Analysis and Public Health

T0074784

This volume showcases new approaches to studying public health in traditional and emerging media, suggesting that we need more analyses that focus on the production of media and on power dynamics, as well as studies of audience reception of media messages.

The collection asks a variety of questions about the role of media in analysing public health. Contributors ask: who is influential in producing the stories we see in the press and on social media? Who benefits, and who is damaged, by media debates on health topics? They investigate the role of big business in seeking to shape public opinion and consumption in print and online media; how issues such as hand washing come to be framed over time by newspapers; how conflicts over immunisations get covered; how health promotion messages do their work; and the positive role of online media in helping foster drug safety. Together, they reach the conclusion that since mass media is a crucial element of civic society, more in-depth understanding of how it works and what impacts it has on public health is essential.

Given the crucial role of the media in shaping health debates, pushing certain issues up the policy agenda, defining problems for audiences and presenting potential solutions, this book's analysis will be of interest to all those studying how the media shape policy, as well as public health researchers with an interest in mass communication. This book was originally published as a special issue of *Critical Public Health*.

Lesley Henderson is a Sociologist and Senior Lecturer in Social and Political Sciences at Brunel University, UK. Her expertise is in communications and social change, and she has published widely on media and public health, science and environmental communication.

Shona Hilton is Deputy Director of the MRC/CSO Social and Public Health Sciences Unit and co-leads a research programme on public health policy at the University of Glasgow, UK. Her research focuses on macro level determinants of public health and the framing of policy debates through scientific, political and media channels.

Judith Green is Professor of Sociology of Health in the School of Population and Environmental Sciences at King's College London, UK, where she co-directs the Social Science and Urban Public Health Institute.

Media Analysis and Public Health

Contemporary Issues in Critical Public Health

Edited by
Lesley Henderson, Shona Hilton
and Judith Green

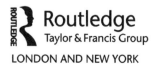

Routledge
Taylor & Francis Group

LONDON AND NEW YORK

First published 2020 by Routledge

2 Park Square, Milton Park, Abingdon, Oxon, OX14 4RN
605 Third Avenue, New York, NY 10017

Routledge is an imprint of the Taylor & Francis Group, an informa business

First issued in paperback 2020

British Library Cataloguing in Publication Data
A catalogue record for this book is available from the British Library

ISBN13: 978-0-367-33598-4 (hbk)
ISBN13: 978-0-367-78454-6 (pbk)

Typeset in Myriad Pro
by Newgen Publishing UK

Publisher's Note
The publisher accepts responsibility for any inconsistencies that may have arisen during the
conversion of this book from journal articles to book chapters, namely the inclusion
of journal terminology.

Disclaimer
Every effort has been made to contact copyright holders for their permission to reprint
material in this book. The publishers would be grateful to hear from any copyright holder
who is not here acknowledged and will undertake to rectify any errors or omissions in future
editions of this book.

Contents

Citation Information

The following chapters were originally published in *Critical Public Health*, volume 28, issue 4 (September 2018). When citing this material, please use the original page numbering for each article, as follows:

Editorial
The media and public health: where next for critical analysis?
Lesley Henderson and Shona Hilton
Critical Public Health, volume 28, issue 4 (September 2018) pp. 373–376

Chapter 1
How the food, beverage and alcohol industries presented the Public Health Responsibility Deal in UK print and online media reports
Nick Douglas, Cecile Knai, Mark Petticrew, Elizabeth Eastmure, Mary Alison Durand and Nicholas Mays
Critical Public Health, volume 28, issue 4 (September 2018) pp. 377–387

Chapter 2
Public engagement and the role of the media in post-marketing drug safety: the case of Eltroxin® (levothyroxine) in New Zealand
Kevin Dew, John Gardner, Elaine H. Morrato, Pauline Norris, Kerry Chamberlain, Darrin Hodgetts and Jonathan Gabe
Critical Public Health, volume 28, issue 4 (September 2018) pp. 388–401

Chapter 3
How alcohol marketing engages users with alcohol brand content on Facebook: an Indian and Australian perspective
Himanshu Gupta, Simone Pettigrew, Tina Lam and Robert J. Tait
Critical Public Health, volume 28, issue 4 (September 2018) pp. 402–411

Chapter 4
'To drink or not to drink': media framing of evidence and debate about alcohol consumption in pregnancy
Kerry McCallum and Kate Holland
Critical Public Health, volume 28, issue 4 (September 2018) pp. 412–423

For any permission-related enquiries please visit:
www.tandfonline.com/page/help/permissions

Notes on Contributors

Crystal Adams is an Assistant Professor of Sociology at Muhlenberg College, USA.

Mary Breheny is an Associate Professor in the School of Health Sciences at Massey University, New Zealand.

Kerry Chamberlain is a Professor of Social and Health Psychology in the School of Psychology at Massey University, New Zealand.

Shefali Chaukra has been affiliated with the School of Public Health and Community Medicine in the Faculty of Medicine at the University of New South Wales, Australia.

Shona Helen Crabb is a Senior Lecturer in the School of Public Health at the University of Adelaide, Australia.

Kevin Dew is a Professor in the School of Social and Cultural Studies at Victoria University of Wellington, New Zealand.

Nick Douglas is a Research Fellow in the Faculty of Public Health and Policy in the Policy Innovation Research Unit at the London School of Hygiene and Tropical Medicine, UK.

Mary Alison Durand is an Associate Professor and Deputy Department Research Degree Co-ordinator in the Department of Health Services Research and Policy at the London School of Hygiene and Tropical Medicine, UK.

Elizabeth Eastmure is an Honorary Research Fellow in the Faculty of Public Health and Policy in the Policy Innovation Research Unit at the London School of Hygiene and Tropical Medicine, UK.

Jonathan Gabe is a Professor of Sociology at the Centre for Criminology and Sociology and in the School of Law at Royal Holloway, University of London, UK.

John Gardner is Health and Biofutures Research Fellow in the School of Social Sciences at Monash University, Australia.

Judith Green is Professor of Sociology in the School of Population and Environmental Sciences at King's College London, UK, where she co-directs the Social Science and Public Health Institute.

Himanshu Gupta is a Research Officer at Menzies School of Health Research, Australia.

Brittany M. Harder is Assistant Professor of Sociology in the Department of History, Sociology, Geography and Legal Studies at the University of Tampa, USA.

Lesley Henderson is a Sociologist and Senior Lecturer in Social and Political Sciences at Brunel University, UK.

Anita Heywood is an Associate Professor in the School of Public Health and Community Medicine in the Faculty of Medicine at the University of New South Wales, Australia.

Shona Hilton is Deputy Director of the MRC/CSO Social and Public Health Sciences Unit and co-leads a research programme on public health policy at the University of Glasgow, UK.

Darrin Hodgetts is a Professor of Societal Psychology in the School of Psychology at Massey University, New Zealand.

Katherine Hodgetts is a Postdoctoral Research Fellow in the School of Public Health at the University of Adelaide, Australia.

Kate Holland is a Senior Research Fellow in Communication and Media Studies in the Faculty of Arts and Design at the University of Canberra, Australia.

Charlotte Bredahl Jacobsen is Director at Virtus, which provides virtual education for students with school absence in Denmark.

Ilan Katz is a Professor at the Social Policy Research Centre at the University of New South Wales, Australia.

Cecile Knai is Assistant Professor of Public Health Policy in the Faculty of Public Health and Policy at the London School of Hygiene and Tropical Medicine, UK.

Dorthe Brogård Kristensen is Associate Professor in the Department of Marketing and Management at the University of Southern Denmark, Denmark.

Tina Lam is a Research Fellow at the Monash Addiction Research Centre (MARC) at Monash University, Australia.

Nicholas Mays is a Professor of Health Policy in the Faculty of Public Health and Directs the Policy in the Policy Innovation Research Unit at the London School of Hygiene and Tropical Medicine, UK.

Kerry McCallum is an Associate Professor in Communication and a Senior Research Fellow in the News and Media Research Centre at the University of Canberra, Australia.

Elaine H. Morrato is an Associate Professor in the Colorado School of Public Health at the University of Colorado Anschutz Medical Campus, USA.

Pauline Norris is a Professor in the School of Pharmacy at the University of Otago, New Zealand.

Mark Petticrew is Professor of Public Health Evaluation in the Faculty of Public Health and Policy at the London School of Hygiene and Tropical Medicine, UK.

Simone Pettigrew is a Distinguished Research Professor in the School of Psychology in the Faculty of Health Sciences at Curtin University, Australia.

Signe Pihl-Thingvad is an Associate Professor in the Department of Political Science and Public Management at the University of Southern Denmark, Denmark.

Christina Severinsen is a Senior Lecturer of Public Health in the School of Health Sciences at Massey University, New Zealand.

Niamh Stephenson is an Associate Professor in Social Science in the School of Public Health and Community Medicine in the Faculty of Medicine at the University of New South Wales, Australia.

Robert J. Tait is a Senior Research Fellow in the Faculty of Health Sciences at the National Drug Research Institute at Curtin University, Australia.

Emma Whelan is Associate Professor in the Department of Sociology and Social Anthropology at Dalhousie University, Canada.

Preface: Media, Evidence and Debate

This is a timely point to consider new directions in critical public health scholarship on the media. There are urgent policy questions around how health issues are covered in the mass media, and with what consequences: immunisation is a good example. Political problems – such as urban violence or climate emergencies – have gained renewed traction with efforts to frame them as 'public health' issues. Debates around these have generated broader scrutiny of how public health communities communicate with the public, and to what effect. One key issue has been how this communication is shaped by other social actors, whose interests may not be aligned with those of public health. Following on from studies of how the tobacco industry strategically sought to shape public opinion through the manufacture of uncertainty and doubt, scholars have turned their attention to other 'harmful commodity' industry players, such as the alcohol and soda industries, and their engagements with the mass media. Scholarship has had to adapt to the context of a rapidly changing landscape of what counts as 'the media'. Form and content have shifted radically with rising use of social media and digital platforms, and arguably a declining role for traditional newsprint. We are only just beginning to understand how these change relationships between health professionals and the public. How have these new forms changed communication style and flows? How have they transformed audience reach, engagement and reception in relation to health knowledge? How are different kinds of expertise legitimised, or undermined, across different platforms? And what kinds of health identities are forged online? Technological change has also generated new research approaches, offering methods for analysing large datasets of micro-encounters with digital media, such as tweets, likes or page visits, and new channels for researchers to directly reach public audiences through online media. Critical public health practice has to better understand how media works in a globalising, digital age – and where the possibilities for change lie.

Mass media, in their changing forms, remain a core component of any health system, providing communication channels and framing health care problems and their solutions. Public health policy makers and practitioners have no choice but to engage with the media. We have to better understand how media messages relate to knowledge, practice, debate and political action, and better understand how to contribute to public debate in ways that are most likely to lead to health and equity gain. However, how to engage is not obvious. The relationships between media coverage of health issues, public knowledge and policy change are never straightforward: there is no simple way in which evidence translates to a message, and then into action. The fault lines of evidence-making, unanticipated consequences of communication strategies and the politics of framing, may be most obvious around issues where health goals come into conflict with those of big business, but they impact across all health domains. Public health does not speak with a monolithic voice: there are debates within public health, and the consequences of policy are rarely straightforwardly healthy or unhealthy – the gains and losses fall differently across global societies. As the chapters in this book show, on topics as diverse as hand-washing, adverse drug reactions, smoking, corporate responsibility, immunisation and social isolation, there is no inevitable way in which evidence, media coverage, public interests and health or equity gains coalesce.

However, the relationships between health concerns and media messages are not of course entirely unpredictable. They are structured by social and political relations. Critical public health scholars have a rich tradition of analysing media texts to demonstrate their discursive effects, and of unpacking how particular health issues get framed within media accounts through systematic relations of power. The first aim of this collection is to showcase these approaches and generate an agenda for key questions for media analysis in public health. The second aim is to stimulate more research on media production. Media coverage does not just arise from a black box, to which more or less powerful other actors make inputs; rather, it is actively produced through particular networks and practices. As Lesley Henderson and Shona Hilton argue in their Introduction, this 'political economy' of media production deserves far greater scrutiny from critical scholars than it has had to date. Our third aim is that the chapters here foster a greater sophistication in relation to media analysis in critical public health. Several authors point to the ways in which 'the media' cannot be simplistically held as responsible for creating public knowledge, misrepresenting evidence or amplifying public concern. Diverse publics are not empty vessels, awaiting messages from a media entirely captured by big business. Publics, like professionals, do not speak with one voice, and are active agents in shaping the contours of public debate – if, often, with rather less access to voice than corporate or state actors. The mass media are a route for mobilising concerns and values, and for creating publics. They are therefore an essential route of critical communication back to the institutions of public health. The research represented here shows the value of this kind of critical, reflexive engagement with how the mass media relates to public health. This should interrogate the role and political economy of the media, but not take relations or effects for granted.

Judith Green
King's College London

Introduction

The media and public health: Where next for critical analysis?

Lesley Henderson and Shona Hilton

In this editorial, we examine what we see as the critical issues facing media research in emerging public health debates and call for a research agenda that takes account of media production, underpinned by political sciences.

It has been well established that the media play a crucial role in framing public health debates and shaping public perceptions by selecting which issues are reported and how they are represented (Seale, 2002). We know that in public health debates, the media contribute to the framing of health problems, their drivers and potential solutions, with stakeholders variously positioned across those debates (Elliot-Green et al., 2016). This is particularly the case when corporate interests run counter to public health interests. In such cases, the media have an important function as both producer of narratives and as narrator to public audiences. However, all too often, the actual processes of media production are absent from analysis – yet these can be vital to consider, as they call into question issues of how culture, power and the political economy influence the debate.

In this respect, media production needs to be considered in its broadest terms, not simply as 'discourse' manufactured in newsrooms, television studios and other media institutions, but as the outcome of specific networks, occupational practices, technologies and structural contexts with embedded ideological assumptions (Henderson, 2018a). As sociologist Stuart Hall argued, the production of meaning or signification within the media narrative is itself a specific practice rather than a mere reflection of reality. Narrative discourses thus become a field in which political and cultural articulations are played out in an attempt to establish hegemonic formations (Hall, 1985). In other words, we need to explore the practice whereby a particular and specific world view becomes the accepted cultural norm.

Non-communicable diseases (NCDs) have been identified as one of the main global public health challenges of the twenty-first century, driven in part by unhealthy commodity industries (Freudenberg, 2014). Despite this, media research in public health has not been able to shed light on comparative media strategies employed by industries marketing commodities such as alcohol, tobacco and ultra-processed foods and beverages that increase NCD risk or how media coverage of these industries influences public health policy debates (Weishaar et al., 2016). In the case of NCDs, media production research could usefully consider the relationships between powerful institutions such as media corporations and the harmful commodity industries driving NCDs. This gap in media research limits our understanding of the detrimental impact of commercial interests on public health and of how best to counter the claims and strategies of such industries when they 'directly lobby' the public and policymakers via the media. Every day, people are bombarded with messages from stakeholders involved in politically contested public health debates. These range from sugar-sweetened beverage taxation, to minimum pricing for alcohol (Hilton, Wood, Patterson, & Katikireddi, 2014), to emerging debates such as the polluting nature of plastics (Henderson, 2018b).

We also know that stakeholders seek to present evidence and arguments for or against specific policy initiatives that are in line with their interests and that they deliberately engage with the media to influence the political climate and promote positive public perceptions of their activities to advance their business goals. Strategies might thus include making 'their' industry goals appear to be 'our' universal goals which are 'naturally' in everyone's interests. For example, promoting the idea that people should be free to choose what they eat, regardless of how healthy their choice, can successfully sideline powerful concerns regarding the global marketing practices of Big Food (for examples, see Williams & Nestle, 2015).

By ignoring the political economy shaping such media discourses, we risk neglecting crucial questions of power and (re)producing media analyses that merely describe health topics in the public domain but fail to reveal the insidious nature of media production in these contexts or to identify strategies for public health advocates. Methodological innovation and engagement with alternative theoretical paradigms can be gained through working with political scientists. New opportunities could be facilitated by a greater focus on comparative research on the representations of different industries whose products increase NCD risk. Current media research tends to focus on describing media representations of single issues or specific topics; however, there may be benefits to appraising media reporting on a range of issues to facilitate learning that transcends individual topics. Analysing debates concerning different public health issues enables identification of key discursive components of policy debates to make some comparisons. A key challenge here is the direct lobbying of the public by industries which have extensive resources to use media in ways which are favourable to their interests. In this special issue, for instance, Douglas, Knai, Eastmure, Durand, & Mays (2018) provide a cross industry focus by examining how the food, beverage and alcohol industries frame public health policy problems and solutions in terms of their own vested interests, demonstrating the sheer reach of industry, legitimising their viewpoints and protecting their agendas.

The role of industry is also of central concern to US sociologists Adams and Harder (2018), who analyse how the pharmaceutical industry constructs lifestyle behaviour in direct-to-consumer television advertising aimed at overweight and obese people by emphasising the necessity of drug regimens to manage health and, in so doing, establish the hegemonic formation of 'being thin' as the desirable norm.

So, in this special media and critical public health issue, we bring together a range of papers from academics and health practitioners based in Australia, India, Canada, the USA, New Zealand, Denmark and the UK. These report on studies which highlight different traditional and 'new' media and explore how public health messaging in the various sites of social media, online news and radio might frame health issues and the ways in which audiences or users engage (or not) with messages. Media reporting both reflects and shapes cultural ideas about public health issues and, perhaps more importantly, frames solutions and responsibilities in ways which are politically charged and have policy consequences. Mass media health campaigns can reach large numbers of people quickly and relatively cheaply, but their efficacy is often critiqued on the grounds that the focus is on individual 'choices' and behaviour, thus obscuring or marginalising power dynamics. We argue here that media are part of the macro factors which influence health behaviour and policy and so critical public health researchers with an interest in media need to ask some key questions such as who is setting the agenda?', 'in whose interests does it serve?' and indeed 'who are the media?'.

Mass media work perhaps most productively where the focus is on life-style health promotion, but has a less clear role for public health issues stemming from social and material conditions. In this issue for example, Whelan (2018) explores how analysis of media reporting might act as a useful lens to view shifts in responsibility and accountability concerning handwashing to curb epidemics. Campaigns where members of the public are encouraged to compel their healthcare provider to wash their hands not only are lacking in efficacy but also fail to take account of power relations and structural constraints because handwashing is linked to inequalities rather than a simple question of individual choice.

Health messaging to promote the daily intake of fruits and vegetables has long been a staple of the traditional mass media public health campaign. Kristensen, Jacobsen, and Pihl-Thingvad (2018) draw on the sociology of quantification to highlight how numbers create scientific legitimacy and authority in diverse audiences. Thus, the social meaning of '6 a day' becomes open to translation: different actors can mobilise discourses which may be different from, and indeed possibly undermine, those of the health communicators, augmenting the message in ways that are difficult to predict.

What we consume in terms of health advertising and how we access health-related messages have changed immeasurably through, for instance, niche personalised media consumption or micro-targeted health advertising. Popular social media such as Facebook offer tremendous possibilities for analysing audiences'/users' engagement with public health messages yet also potentially open up new spaces in which powerful industries might circumvent codes of practice, targeting younger audiences who may be unaware of the pernicious nature of alcohol marketing. As Gupta, Pettigrew, Lam, and Tait (2018) highlight, this form of marketing is flexible and user-focused: it can be adapted to suit the preferences of consumers, albeit without their knowledge, offering fresh challenges for regulation.

However, it is crucial that we do not fall into traps of simple moral panics concerning the role of new media in public health. Indeed, the study of media and post-marketing drug safety in New Zealand, by Dew et al. (2018), highlights how media reporting can play a key role in increased pharmacovigilance, in which patients report adverse drug reactions. Here, the authors argue that such increased reporting should not be dismissed as just another media fuelled 'health scare', but instead drug safety agencies should be tracking and engaging with (social) media to follow up on post-marketing concerns.

Media advocacy groups now commonly work closely with journalists to engender trust and credibility for public health messages. Stephenson, Chaukra, and Heywood (2018) demonstrate how, in Australia, media framing of the single issue of immunisation can reveal important ambiguities within public health regarding the positioning of parents and why it is important to move beyond the binary 'pro' and 'anti' stance.

There has been a significant body of research which has highlighted a consistent media focus on gender and the body. This is intensified with media stories of pregnancy and public health messages regarding smoking and alcohol. Here, women are 'policed' and under intense surveillance. McCallum and Holland (2018) analyse pregnancy and parenting websites and news stories identifying how drinking during pregnancy was framed as an issue of 'women's rights', thus potentially introducing ambiguity into a simple Australian Government message of abstinence. In a similarly themed paper, the rise of the non-professional actor through reality television, a relatively recent phenomenon, highlights the intense media interest in celebrity 'motherhood'. Hodgetts and Crabb (2018) conduct a discourse analysis of an Australian media personality who is shamed and forced to 'confess' to smoking during pregnancy.

Breheny and Severinsen (2018) shed light on the reporting of social isolation amongst older people, which is framed rightly within public health as an issue with profound health implications. The authors analyse online interactions concerning these stories and found, however, that the issue was reframed as a consequence of "poor choices" and family 'inadequacy'. This raises important issues regarding the uncritical celebration of online public forums being a democratising 'healthy' space.

We are thus calling for more holistic approaches to media studies that build upon overarching questions that fully engage with the changing nature of 'the media'. With the advent of Web 2.0, images, videos and text are produced daily, representing almost every topic of interest to public health researchers. This brings new methodological challenges in how to analyse the content of these media communications. So we are asking, in our current increasingly complex environment, what are the challenges for critical public health and how can engaging with media in a critical fashion help shed light on power dynamics that underpin these relationships? We call for a critical media analysis which takes account of the complexity of our media saturated contemporary landscape, which shifts away from individualistic case studies and linear models of power that implies the 'dissemination' of health messages to 'the public'. Instead, we should build and draw upon theoretical frameworks developed in sociology, media and cultural studies, which may also overlap with a rich literature concerning public understandings of science, health and science communication

References

Adams, C., & Harder, B. M. (2018). Diet, exercise…*and* drugs: Social constructions of healthy lifestyles in weight-related prescription drug advertisements. *Critical Public Health, 28*(4), 439–449.

Breheny, M., & Severinsen, C. (2018). Is social isolation a public health issue? A media analysis in Aotearoa/New Zealand. *Critical Public Health, 28*(4), 484–493.

Dew, K., Gardner, J., Morrato, E. H., Norris, P., Chamberlain, K., & Hodgetts, D. (2018). Public engagement and the role of the media in post-marketing drug safety: The case of Eltroxin® (levothyroxine) in New Zealand. *Critical Public Health, 28*(4), 388–401.

Douglas, N., Knai, C., Eastmure, E., Durand, M. A., & Mays, N. (2018). How the food, beverage and alcohol industries presented the Public Health Responsibility Deal in UK print and online media reports. *Critical Public Health, 28*(4), 377–387.

Elliott-Green, A., Hyseni, L., Lloyd-Williams, F., Bromley, H., & Capewell, S. (2016). Sugar-sweetened beverages coverage in the British media: An analysis of public health advocacy versus pro-industry messaging. *BMJ Open, 6*(7).

Freudenberg, N. (2014). *Lethal but legal. corporations, consumption and protecting public health.* New York: Oxford University Press.

Gupta, H., Pettigrew, S., Lam, T., & Tait, R. J. (2018). How alcohol marketing engages users with alcohol brand content on Facebook: An Indian and Australian perspective. *Critical Public Health, 28*(4), 402–411.

Hall, S. (1985). The rediscovery of 'ideology': Return of the repressed in media studies. In V. Beechey & J. Donald (Eds.), *Subjectivity and social relations* (pp. 2–23). Milton Keynes: Open University Press.

Henderson, L. (2018a). Popular television and public mental health: Creating media entertainment from mental distress. *Critical Public Health, 28*(1), 106–117.

Henderson, L. (2018b). *Solving the problem of plastic pollution: Beyond the natural sciences?* (Cost of Living). Retrieved May 25, 2018, from https://www.cost-ofliving.net/solving-the-problem-of-plastic-pollution-beyond-the-natural-sciences/

Hilton, S., Wood, K., Patterson, C., & Katikireddi, S. V. (2014). Implications for alcohol minimum unit pricing advocacy: What can we learn for public health from UK newsprint coverage of key claim-makers in the policy debate? *Social Science & Medicine, 102*, 157–164.

Hodgetts, K., & Crabb, S. H. (2018). 'I cannot explain it. I knew it was wrong': A public account of cigarette smoking in pregnancy. *Critical Public Health, 28*(4), 450–459.

Kristensen, D. B., Jacobsen, C. B., & Pihl-Thingvad, S. (2018). Perception and translation of numbers: The case of a health campaign in Denmark. *Critical Public Health, 28*(4), 460–471.

McCallum, K., & Holland, K. (2018). To drink or not to drink': Media framing of evidence and debate about alcohol consumption in pregnancy. *Critical Public Health, 28*(4), 412–423.

Seale, C. (2002). *Media and health.* London: SAGE Publications.

Stephenson, N., Chaukra, S., & Heywood, A. (2018). Newspaper coverage of childhood immunisation in Australia: A lens into conflicts within public health. *Critical Public Health, 28*(4), 472–483.

Weishaar, H., Dorfman, L., Freudenberg, N., Hawkins, B., Smith, K., Razum, O., et al. (2016). Why media representations of corporations matter for public health policy: A scoping review. *BMC Public Health, 16*, 899.

Whelan, E. (2018). Working up a lather: The rise (and fall?) of hand hygiene in Canadian newspapers, 1986–2015. *Critical Public Health, 28*(4), 424–438.

Williams, S., & Nestle, M. (2015). 'Big food': Taking a critical perspective on a global public health problem. *Critical Public Health, 25*, 245–247.

Lesley Henderson

http://orcid.org/0000-0002-0317-2890

Shona Hilton

http://orcid.org/0000-0003-0633-8152

1 How the food, beverage and alcohol industries presented the Public Health Responsibility Deal in UK print and online media reports

Nick Douglas, Cecile Knai, Mark Petticrew, Elizabeth Eastmure, Mary Alison Durand and Nicholas Mays

ABSTRACT

The Public Health Responsibility Deal (RD) in England is a public–private partnership between government, industry and other stakeholders aiming to improve public health in four key areas: food, alcohol, health at work and physical activity. Wider literature shows that industry engages in framing of public health policy problems, solutions and its role in solutions that is favourable to its interests. As part of an evaluation of the RD, we conducted a media analysis to explore how industry spokespersons (from commercial enterprises, trade associations and social aspects/public relations organisations) represented the RD in newspaper and online reports. We systematically searched databases indexing articles of British national newspapers and the online news services of national broadcasters for articles published between 2010 and 2015. After application of inclusion criteria, we identified 247 relevant articles. We extracted direct quotations by industry spokespersons and analysed them thematically. Media reporting about the RD provided industry spokespersons with a high-profile platform to present frames relating to food, beverages and alcohol that were favourable to advancing or protecting industry positions and agendas. Framing of issues addressed responsibility for public health problems, policy options and the role of industry, also legitimising industry spokespersons to advocate a position on how public health policy should evolve. Media analysis can elucidate industry discourses around public health and examine their engagement in framing to extend their influence in public health policy.

Introduction

The Public Health Responsibility Deal (RD) was launched in 2011 as a public–private partnership consisting of voluntary agreements between government, industry and other stakeholders in England aiming to improve public health (Department of Health, 2011). Signatories pledge to undertake public health-related activity as part of four networks: food, alcohol, health at work and physical activity.

Media reports can play a crucial role in selecting issues for public attention, policy agenda setting, framing issues in a particular way and shaping perceptions about who is responsible for social problems (Kim & Willis, 2007). Framing is an integral technique of media reporting. It can function to enable the construction of meaning and the provision of a logic that renders an issue comprehensible; shape the parameters of a public policy debate (i.e. problem definition, causal attribution, recommended remedial action); identify an issue or problem as political in nature; identify legitimate participants/ commentators; and open up some policy options/solutions while closing down others (Hawkins & Holden, 2013; Nixon et al., 2015).

Studies have identified how alcohol, food and beverage industries engage in framing to influence public discourse about public health problems, solutions and the role of industry in those solutions that is favourable to their interests (Brownell & Warner, 2009; Casswell, 2013; Hawkins & Holden, 2013; Mialon, Swinburn, & Sacks, 2015). Hawkins and Holden (2013), drawing on Snow and Benford (1988) and Benford and Snow (2000), offer a useful conceptual schema for understanding framing activity by industry actors: *diagnostic framing* seeks to define the problems, *prognostic framing* offers solutions to the problems identified and *motivational framing* seeks to enlist support and move people to act to effect social change.

As part of a larger, independent evaluation of the RD commissioned by the English Department of Health in 2013, we conducted a media analysis of public statements in newspaper articles and online news reports by industry spokespersons. The term 'industry' refers here to food and drinks producers, manufacturers, wholesalers, retailers, trade associations and social aspects/public relations organisa- tions funded by relevant industries (Babor, 2009). We sought to explore whether and how industry spokespersons framed and presented the RD in ways that protected their commercial interests and promoted core business goals. Our analysis of news reports about the RD examined how industry spokespersons framed the public health challenges the RD was designed to address, their preferred policy solutions and their role as RD partners. We focused on industry spokespersons as industry par- ticipation in the RD was a contentious issue, with the UK Faculty of Public Health withdrawing from the RD and its president stating that industry interests were being prioritised over public health, alongside the withdrawal of a number of non-governmental health organisations (Boseley, 2011; Limb, 2013; Panjwani & Caraher, 2014).

Methods

Searching

We identified print and online news articles containing direct quotations from spokespersons about the RD. Table 1 summarises the process we undertook to search for, screen, code and analyse the articles identified.

During March 2015, we searched for articles published between 31 October 2010 and 28 February 2015 in all national daily newspapers in (mainland) Britain via two newspaper article databases (LexisNexis and ProQuest). This included newspapers reflecting editorial styles ranging across the political spectrum and those that featured longer, in-depth articles as well as those written in a brief, tabloid style. We also searched the websites of three main national television news broadcasters pro- viding online news coverage (*BBC News, Channel 4 News, Sky News*) for the same time period, using each website's search facility. We identified 606 articles in total (see Supplementary Material – Figure 1). Search terms used were 'Public Health Responsibility Deal' or 'responsibility deal'.

Screening

After preliminary screening of database search records to remove duplicates and non-relevant arti- cles, 399 articles remained. Full-text articles were imported into Endnote 7 for data management. Two researchers independently performed a second screening to remove duplicates and those that contained no specific reference to or quotations about the RD. We used the criteria in Table 1 to cate- gorise the articles. After independent categorisation, we identified an initial difference between the two researchers' assessments regarding around 10% of articles. This was resolved in all cases following

Table 1. Methods.

1.1. Summary of methods	
Search	• Dates of searches: March 2015 • Dates of articles: 31/10/10 and 28/2/15 • Search terms: 'Public Health Responsibility Deal' or 'responsibility deal' • Databases searched: LexisNexis and ProQuest • Websites searched: *BBC News, Channel 4 News, Sky News*
Screening	• Full text downloaded to Endnote 7 • Duplicates – removed • Articles with no specific references to the RD – removed • Articles with no quotations about the RD – removed • Two researchers independently screened articles according to selection criteria – see 1.2 • 10% discrepancy in designation of articles identified – resolved following review and discussion without need for review by third researcher
Coding and textual analysis	• Articles categorised 3 or 4 imported into NVivo 10 • Articles read in full • Quotations from each article extracted – name of the speaker and organisational attribution (where given) recorded • Coding conducted according to principles of Braun and Clarke's (2006) approach to thematic analysis by first author • 20% of thematic coding reviewed by second author – no discrepancies identified

1.2. Article categorisation criteria

1. Not substantively about the RD
2. Is about the RD but contains no quotes
3. Not substantively about the RD but does contain quotes about it. (Articles were also ranked 3 where there was reference to the RD but quotes referred to 'voluntary agreements' or where the context made it explicit that the person quoted was referring to the RD even if the specific phrase RD was not used.)
4. Substantively about the RD and contains quotes about the RD

review and discussion so that an agreed classification was reached without need for referral to a third designated researcher. Following this process, 247 articles that were about the RD and/or contained quotations about the RD were identified and imported into NVivo 10 for textual analysis (see Supplementary Material – Figure 1).

Coding and analysis

We read all articles and extracted only text from each article that was clearly identifiable as a direct quotation (we retained additional surrounding text to preserve original context and meaning). The only exceptions were comment pieces by identified authors or letters to the editor, which we treated as extended quotations. The name of the speaker and organisational attribution (where given) were recorded and speakers were grouped by organisational type (see Supplementary Material – Figure 2).

We then reread all quotations in full. The first author then coded and analysed them according to Braun and Clarke's (2006) approach to thematic analysis, using an inductive approach, i.e. generating themes in a grounded way from the data rather than using a priori categories. Examples of coding are provided as illustration (see Supplementary Material – Table 2). The second researcher examined 20% of the thematic coding. No discrepancies were identified.

We then extracted the quotations attributed to industry spokespersons. The data analysed were 83 coded excerpts containing quotations from 68 articles.

A thematic map was generated based on the inductive coding of quotations from these spokespersons, representing the discursive themes deployed (see Supplementary Material – Figure 3). In accordance with the thematic map, we present findings on positive and critical views about the RD by spokespersons quoted; the balance of content in quotations regarding the four RD networks; representations of the public health challenges and the role of industry; preferred policy responses; and reputation enhancement and corporate social responsibility. Articles that featured the quotations presented in the following findings are listed in Supplementary Material –Table 3.

Findings

Data from 21 different newspapers and the online news services of three TV broadcasters were included. Of the 247 articles analysed, the most common sources were *The Guardian* (n = 47, 19%) and *Daily Mail Newspapers* (n = 35, 14%), and *BBC News* online (n = 33, 13%), cumulatively accounting for almost half of the articles analysed (n = 115, 46%) (see Supplementary Material – Figure 4). Of the 218 spokespersons, government (n = 54) and industry (n = 48) representatives were most often quoted, followed by those from NGOs (n = 37) (see Supplementary Material – Figure 2). The findings as follows focus on the analysis of quotations attributed to industry spokespersons.

With the exception of the dissenting voices discussed below, quotations about the RD from industry spokespersons were frequently expressed in positive terms, with phrases such as 'practical, measurable, deliverable', 'positive and progressive work', 'the start of a journey' and 'significant development' used.

> These pledges represent a great start to what we hope will be a long-term shared plan to improve alcohol awareness and reduce alcohol harm. Stefan Orlowski, Heineken (*News of the World*, 2011 March 13).

Although there are four RD networks (food, alcohol, health at work and physical activity), almost all of the quotes concerned food and/or alcohol or referred to the RD and participation in general terms, with very little material regarding the latter two networks. Only two quotes substantively addressed physical activity and health at work, both of which referred to an RD health at work initiative by one alcohol producer.

> 'I'm a really keen cyclist but I decided to go along to the yoga classes at the office to try something new,' he said. 'It's proven to be a brilliant stress buster and I've met new colleagues, which oils the wheels of the working day. Combine this with things like nutrition seminars we attended recently and healthy food in the restaurant, and you feel as though you are being given the tools to help be your best. That's good for me and good for the business too.' Jeff Lawrence – Finance Manager, Pernod Ricard UK Division, (*The Times*, 2013 Jan 01).

The public health challenge

Industry spokespersons acknowledged the RD as a response to concerns about public health problems associated with food and alcohol consumption. However, the arguments presented: (1) downplayed the responsibility of industry for these public health problems, (2) deployed the RD as evidence that industry was sufficiently playing its part, (3) stated that the focus of policy intervention should be the individual consumer and not the activities of industry, (4) advocated the RD as a preferable policy alternative to those that industry opposed.

Downplaying industry responsibility

The first key argument was that industry was not responsible for the public health concerns being addressed by the RD (chiefly focusing in their comments on obesity and alcohol harm). For example, industry spokespersons challenged the link between consumption of high-sugar drinks and obesity, and sought to downplay the responsibility of soft drinks producers.

> Over the last 10 years, the consumption of soft drinks containing added sugar has fallen by 9% while the incidence of obesity has been increasing, and 61% of soft drinks now contain no added sugar. Gavin Partington – Director General, British Soft Drinks Association (*Sky News Online*, 2013 February 18).

Arguments around problems associated with alcohol consumption focused not on population level health harms but on an irresponsible minority of consumers who were reportedly failing to adhere to 'responsible drinking' messages, thus, displacing responsibility from industry to these consumers. This quotation from a letter to the editor responding to an article on minimum unit pricing is illustrative.

> Pushing up the price of alcohol would unfairly penalise the responsible majority of drinkers and hit the poorest hardest, while doing nothing to tackle the root causes of alcohol misuse [...] It is this [RD] partnership working, not MUP, that is the key to tackling the minority that consume alcohol irresponsibly. Miles Beale – Chief Executive, Wine & Spirit Trade Association (*The Daily Telegraph*, 2013 October 02).

Industry already playing its part

The second key argument was that industry was already sufficiently playing its part on a voluntary basis in addressing public health problems as part of a partnership approach. Spokespersons referred to initiatives underway to address obesity and alcohol-related health harms such as clearer food labelling, the RD pledge to reduce a billion units of alcohol produced, reformulation of products to reduce sugar, salt and fat, and the introduction of so-called 'guilt-free lanes' (checkouts free from high fat, high-sugar confectionary).

> UK food and drink manufacturers are keen to do their part [...] demonstrating that voluntary action can deliver in many of these key areas [...] Through the Responsibility Deal, UK food and drink manufacturers are working in partnership with government, non-governmental organisations and other stakeholders to tackle the causes of obesity and poor public health. It is an important part of the UK food manufacturing industry's commitment to achieving responsible and sustainable economic growth. Barbara Gallani – Director of Food Safety, Science and Health, Food and Drink Federation (*Financial Times*, 2012 August 06).

Consumer responsibility not industry regulation

The third key argument was that policy intervention should focus on the individual consumer. This focused on providing information about 'healthy choices' and promoting individual behaviour change.

> The Responsibility Deal is just one part of the government's public health strategy. It is an ongoing process and the public health community can help shape the agenda. I don't believe the public want the way they eat, drink and exercise in their own homes legislated by government. Helping people make better choices has to be a better long-term approach. Jeremy Beadles – Chief Executive, Wine and Spirit Trade Association (*The Guardian*, 2011 February 25).

In the context of alcohol specifically, activity to address the behaviour of the aforementioned irresponsible minority of problem drinkers was advocated through 'responsible drinking' initiatives, thus shifting the emphasis away from examination of industry responsibility towards individuals or, in one instance, 'society'.

> The Government's Responsibility Deal is to be welcomed, and the partnership gives us an opportunity to build on our existing responsible drinking programme. Stefan Orlowski – Managing Director, Heineken UK (*The Sunday Telegraph*, 2011 March 13).

> Clearly, we have to re-educate consumers in such a way that they consume responsibly and encourage their children to do the same. If you get merry as the by-product of an evening, we've all been there; if you set out to get legless before you go out, clearly society has got it wrong. Michael Turner – Executive Chairman, Fullers (*The Daily Telegraph*, 2011 April 27).

Industry spokespersons also opposed increased regulatory measures. Regarding food and alcohol labelling, for example, industry spokespersons suggested that more stringent regulation was either impossible to comply with, counterproductive or unnecessary. Spokesperson's indicated that the space on packaging for further information was too limited; that information was available to consumers through other means if they wanted it (i.e. websites or asking customer services staff) or that hard-hitting messages on alcohol containers might prove counterproductive by making the products more attractive to young people.

> On a small label, we are only able to present a limited amount of information. Anyone interested in understanding the nutritional content with the [salad] dressing can find this on our website or speak to any of our team in the shop, who have this information readily to hand. Anonymous Spokesperson, Eat [Fast Food Chain] (*Daily Mail*, 2014 October 06).

> She told the BBC News channel that 'graphic' health warnings on alcohol packaging would be a 'step too far'. 'I think there's lots of information out there for people. The industry here is doing incredible amounts of work in terms of voluntarily putting the government's guidelines on alcohol. Just look at the back of your label and you'll see things like the number of units in there, the chief medical officer's guidelines and all sorts of other useful information out there for consumers.' Sarah Hanratty – Deputy Chief Executive, Portman Group (*BBC News Online*, 2014 August 11).

The RD as a policy alternative

Significantly, the fourth key argument was to propose the RD as preferable to policies opposed by industry – regulation, mandatory product labelling or fiscal mechanisms, such as minimum unit pricing on alcohol and taxation on high-sugar products, particularly soft drinks.

> The BSDA's Director General Gavin Partington said 61% of soft drinks 'now contain no added sugar and we have seen soft drinks companies lead the way in committing to further, voluntary action as part of the government's Responsibility Deal calorie-reduction pledge.' He said 10p from every 60p can of drink already goes to the government in tax. 'Putting up taxes even further will put pressure on people's purses at a time when they can ill afford it,' he said. Gavin Partington – Director General, British Soft Drinks Association (*BBC News Online*, 2013 January 29).

> The intended introduction of [minimum unit] pricing intervention is misguided and appears to run counter to the Responsibility Deal set out by this government. Andrew Cowan – Director, Diageo GB (*BBC News* Online, 2012 March 23).

There was an explicit recognition from one spokesperson that participation in the RD might be a strategically useful response on the part of industry to resist calls for regulatory policy responses from government.

> The Association of Licensed Multiple Retailers has told members: 'Ministers have made it clear that signing up to the deal will be taken into account in considering new legislation in these areas. This could help fend off further calls for action from the health lobby.' Anonymous Spokesperson – Association of Licensed Multiple Retailers (*The Daily Telegraph*, 2011 March 12).

The role of industry

Given the centrality of the notion of partnership to the RD, it was important to understand how industry spokespersons discussed and framed the role of industry. There were two key themes: that involvement of industry was the optimal solution as part of a partnership approach to the public health challenges discussed, and that there was a legitimate role for industry in formulating public health policy on these issues.

For example, spokespersons indicated that involving industry represented the most viable and pragmatic approach to tackling the public health problems that the RD was designed to address. The key themes that informed this argument were that industry had a specialist body of knowledge, expertise and experience, plus the ability to reach the public, such that failing to involve them would miss an important opportunity.

> It is precisely the leading brands like PepsiCo that have the reach, resources and marketing capabilities to influence the diets of hundreds of thousands of people in the UK. The government has chosen to recognise this and harness industry knowledge by introducing the Responsibility Deal [...] How about we are brought inside so that our influence over people's diets can be used positively to promote healthier eating? I think the government, by including food companies in its Responsibility Deal, has made the right choice. Richard Evans – President, PepsiCo (*BBC News* Online, 2011 March 15).

Another similar line of argument was that the public health challenges faced (i.e. obesity and alcohol-related health problems) were too complex for government or health bodies to tackle alone and that only a private–public partnership could work.

> A complex, multi-faceted problem like alcohol abuse requires a comprehensive, multi-faceted response – and that is what the Public Health Responsibility Deal provides. It sets out practical, measurable and deliverable steps which can be a real catalyst for change if everyone plays their part. Sue Clark – Director of Corporate Affairs, SABMiller (*BBC News* Online, 2011 March 20).

Comment from one spokesperson suggested that industry had not only a responsibility to contribute its expertise but a right to be involved in public health policy-making as an equal stakeholder alongside others.

> At Diageo we believe we have a responsibility to share our knowledge of operating in this sector, and that we have a right to be heard – just like any other stakeholder. We are but one voice, one perspective, alongside NGOs, academics, the medical community, the police, politicians and consumers. The Responsibility Deal is an excellent example of how a collaborative approach, with every interest represented, can work. Simon Litherland – Managing Director, Diageo GB (*The Guardian*, 2011 February 19).

Reputational enhancement and corporate social responsibility

Industry spokespersons were explicit about the reputational and CSR benefits of participation in the RD. This was stated as potentially good for profitability.

> Our customers expect us to do the right thing. Our pledges to remove alcohol from the entrance of our stores and invest £1 m to tackle alcohol misuse by young people are part of our broader health agenda. Andy Clarke – Chief Executive Officer, Asda (*The Sunday Telegraph*, 2011 March 13).

> Sainsbury's Director of Corporate Affairs, Alex Cole, says what is good for our waistline is also good for the company's bottom-line. 'There's absolutely a business case for doing this. We know our customers want products that are healthier. If we can provide them with those options, an easy way for them to make a healthy choice, we do sell more.' Alex Cole – Director of Corporate Affairs, Sainsbury's (*Sky News Online*, 2013 October 26).

Dissenting voices

Our analysis also sought to identify dissenting voices from those supporting the RD. Although the balance of commentary was strongly oriented towards welcoming and championing the RD, there were instances where even voluntary RD initiatives were described as an inappropriate intervention into what should be private and personal matters.

> The Department of Health's Public Health Responsibility Deal has pledges from the big drinks businesses to reduce the amount drunk in Britain by 1 billion units by the end of 2015. Smith is worried that the 'nanny state' will step in: 'Supermarkets and bars will be flooded with low ABV crap. We don't need government interference. They want to take away our happy juice.' Claire Smith – Head of Spirit Creation, Belvedere Vodka (*The Sunday Times*, 2014 June 08).

> The [Health at Work] pledge on young people [...] obliges employers to 'assume a level of responsibility for the behaviour of employees that intrudes into their personal lives'. He adds: 'We are not their parents; we are a business.' Ralph Findlay – Chief Executive, Marston's (*The Times*, 2012 June 26).

Discussion

Main findings

The news media quotations analysed as part of this study primarily addressed the most contentious health policy issues focused on within the RD namely, food (and by extension obesity) and alcohol consumption. Attention to health at work and physical activity was almost entirely absent. It is interesting to speculate on what accounts for the relative lack of media attention to the latter two networks. It may be the case that editors and journalists regarded these issues as simply less 'newsworthy'.

Despite a small minority of dissenting views founded on concerns about 'nanny-statism', the RD was portrayed as wholeheartedly welcomed by industry and reportedly played an explicit part in CSR agendas.

Media stories provided industry with a platform in the public domain to frame debates about public health in the context of the RD. Referring to Hawkins' and Holden's schema on framing (2013), the diagnostic frame deployed by industry spokespersons resisted their accountability for public health problems and framed the issues as ones of personal responsibility of individual consumers (Brownell & Warner, 2009; Miller & Harkins, 2010; Moodie et al., 2013; Savell, Fooks, & Gilmore, 2016) or an irresponsible minority, thus deflecting attention from the potential contribution of industry (Alcohol Focus Scotland, 2013; Casswell, 2013; Hawkins, Holden, & McCambridge, 2012; Savell et al., 2016).

The prognostic frame deployed proposed that industry was taking sufficient voluntary action on public health problems and used the RD to counter calls for more interventionist forms of government action – despite criticism and little evidence of the health benefits of such public–private partnerships (Moodie et al., 2013; Panjwani & Caraher, 2014; Savell et al., 2016). Instead, individualised policy interventions with the weakest evidence of effectiveness were advocated (consumer education and self-regulation), while those known to have the best evidence of effectiveness were attacked (regulation, price control and marketing control) (Alcohol Focus Scotland, 2013; Hawkins et al., 2012; Miller, de Groot, McKenzie, & Droste, 2011).

Motivational framing argued that the policy-making arena needed to be made more accessible to industry because of its reported expertise and ability to reach the public. The promotion of partnership working appeared to be designed to extend influence and claims for legitimacy of industrial interests (Alcohol Focus Scotland, 2013; Freedhoff & Hebert, 2011; Hawkins et al., 2012; Moodie et al., 2013; Savell et al., 2016). This also implicitly extended industry's claims to expertise beyond food and beverage manufacture, retail and marketing into the realms of population health and public health policy (Moodie et al., 2013; Savell et al., 2016). Similar findings about the RD as a vehicle to stave off government legislation and the appeal of potential reputation enhancement were separately identified in qualitative interviews with industry participants undertaken elsewhere in our evaluation of the RD (Durand et al., 2015).

Recent analysis of the deployment of arguments by food, beverage, alcohol and gambling industries about the complexity of public health challenges also identified the emergence of a set of frames, described as a cross industry 'playbook' (a strategy initially developed by the tobacco industry and akin to a script identifying 'lines to take', Brownell & Warner, 2009) that allowed them to shape the discourse and align it to industry goals in ways that were contrary to public health. For example, by advancing arguments that consumption of problematic products is declining; that such consumption is only minimally, if at all, a contributor to public health harms; that a problematic minority should be the focus of intervention; that measures such as taxation are ineffective in solving such public health problems, with responsibility placed on the individual consumer (Petticrew et al., 2017). Such arguments were remarkably similar to ones identified in our analysis, such that we can locate our findings in a wider context of industry practice in seeking to influence the debate on public health matters.

Strengths and limitations

Picard and Yeo's (2011) review finds that the literature on media coverage of medical and health issues in the UK is underdeveloped. This study adds to and reinforces the conclusions of previous studies on the framing strategies used by industry in the public health arena by examining the issue through the particular lens of the RD; a significant public health policy in England based on a public–private partnership.

We cannot discount the possibility that some individuals were misquoted or that quotations were misattributed. We also cannot entirely escape the effects of media framing as against industry framing: journalists and editors decided on the theme and content of articles, from whom to seek quotations and how to deploy and edit them. Kim and Willis (2007) have reflected on the tendency of the news media (in the US) to focus on individual explanations and solutions for health problems rather than societal ones. Harrabin, Coote, and Allen's (2003) UK study reported a bias against coverage of public health stories in favour of health service crises stories and health scares, which may have affected how quotations were selected and used.

The inclusion of local newspapers may also have altered our analysis. However, a preliminary scan indicated that local publications tended to reproduce stories generated by national newspapers. Similarly, our analysis might have been altered if it had included 'trade press' or radio and television coverage. We also cannot identify how representative those quoted are of industry perspectives. However, it is clear, based on their job titles and positions that those quoted were senior figures within companies and large corporations, with the likely support or approval of public relations departments and company boards. This analysis also focuses only on quotations from industry spokespersons and there is important further work to be done on the media participation of other key groups regarding public–private partnerships, as well as the contestation of frames by such groups. However, the perspectives of a broader range of key participants have received attention in other analyses conducted as part of the RD evaluation (Durand et al., 2015).

Conclusions

This study demonstrates that media representations can be a useful source of data for understanding food, beverage and alcohol industry participation in public health discourse. Analysis of quotations attributed to (predominantly food and alcohol) industry spokespersons in national newspapers and online articles about the RD identified the framing of issues in ways that was favourable to advancing or protecting industry positions and agendas. This is hardly unexpected. Media reporting allows those quoted to frame the issues in order to shape public perceptions and serve their interests (Nixon et al., 2015). Morrell, Forsyth, Lipworth, Kerridge, and Jordens's (2015) Australian study of journalist engagement with health-related industries identified rising concern in health research that such industries inappropriately influence news content and the possibility that journalists overestimate their ability to resist this process.

Industry is not a disinterested partner in public health. It has been argued that its primary goal is to maximise profit and its ultimate responsibility is to shareholders, creating inherent tensions and potential conflicts of interest (Casswell, 2013; Moodie et al., 2013; Wallack, 1992). One criticism expressed from the outset of the RD by some commentators was that public–private partnership would allow and provide a platform for industry to appropriate public health initiatives to advance or protect its own interests (Hawkins et al., 2012; Panjwani & Caraher, 2014). As Koon, Hawkins, and Mayhew (2016) state '… interpretive research on framing looks at how actors create meaning in the policy process and how they package these meanings for instrumental and expressive purposes. In this way, a frame emerges, interacts with others and helps shape the terrain of the debate (p. 807)'. Our findings suggest that media coverage about the RD provided a high-profile opportunity for industry spokespersons to comment on public health policy related to food, soft drinks and alcohol, enabling them to advocate a legitimised position on how public health policy should evolve (Panjwani & Caraher, 2014), and potentially influence the public debate on these issues. As Hawkins and Holden (2013) conceptualise them (citing Weiss, 1989), frames are 'weapons of advocacy' and Miller and Harkins (2010) have documented how 'media capture' is a central tactic of industry to gain influence in policy-making relating to the regulation of food and drink products. For this reason, close attention to what industry says publicly about public–private partnerships in the context of public health is important.

Acknowledgements

We would like to thank Dr Ben Hawkins from the London School of Hygiene and Tropical Medicine and Dr Hilary Thompson from the University of Glasgow for comments on earlier drafts of this paper. Sole responsibility for this paper lies with the authors.

Disclosure statement

The authors report no conflicts of interest.

Funding

This paper is based on independent research commissioned and funded by the NIHR Policy Research Programme Policy Innovation Research Unit. The views expressed in the publication are those of the authors and not necessarily those of the NHS, the NIHR, the Department of Health and Social Care, arms-length bodies or other government departments. The NIHR played no role in the design of the study, the interpretation of the findings, the writing of the paper, or the decision to submit.

References

Alcohol Focus Scotland. (2013). *Engaging with the alcohol industry: What you need to know*. Scotland. Retrieved from http://www.alcohol-focus-scotland.org.uk/media/60010/Engaging-with-the-alcohol-industry-briefing.pdf

Babor, T. F. (2009). Alcohol research and the alcoholic beverage industry: Issues, concerns and conflicts of interest. *Addiction, 104*(s1), 34–47.

Benford, R. D., & Snow, D. A. (2000). Framing processes and social movements: An overview and assessment. *Annual Review of Sociology, 26*, 611–639.

Boseley, S. (2011, March 15). Charities Refuse to Sign up for Government's Health Drive. *The Guardian*, 12. London.

Braun, V., & Clarke, V. (2006). Using thematic analysis in psychology. *Qualitative Research in Psychology, 3*(2), 77–101.

Brownell, K. D., & Warner, K. E. (2009). The perils of ignoring history: Big tobacco played dirty and millions died. How similar is big food? *Milbank Quarterly, 87*(1), 259–294. doi:10.1111/j.1468-0009.2009.00555.x

Casswell, S. (2013). Vested interests in addiction research and policy. Why do we not see the corporate interests of the alcohol industry as clearly as we see those of the tobacco industry? *Addiction, 108*(4), 680–685.

Department of Health. (2011). *The Public Health Responsibility Deal*. Retrieved from https://responsibilitydeal.dh.gov.uk/wp-content/uploads/2012/03/The-Public-Health-Responsibility-Deal-March-2011.pdf

Durand, M. A., Petticrew, M., Goulding, L., Eastmure, E., Knai, C., & Mays, N. (2015). An evaluation of the Public Health Responsibility Deal: Informants' experiences and views of the development, implementation and achievements of a pledge-based, public–private partnership to improve population health in England. *Health Policy, 119*(11), 1506–1514.

Freedhoff, Y., & Hebert, P. C. (2011). Partnerships between health organizations and the food industry risk derailing public health nutrition. *Canadian Medical Association Journal, 183*(3), 291–292.

Harrabin, R., Coote, A., & Allen, J. (2003). *Health in the news. Risk, reporting and media influence (summary)*. London: The King's Fund.

Hawkins, B., & Holden, C. (2013). Framing the alcohol policy debate: Industry actors and the regulation of the UK beverage alcohol market. *Critical Policy Studies, 7*(1), 53–71. doi:10.1080/19460171.2013.766023

Hawkins, B., Holden, C., & McCambridge, J. (2012). Alcohol industry influence on UK alcohol policy: A new research agenda for public health. *Critical Public Health, 22*(3), 297–305. doi:10.1080/09581596.2012.658027

Kim, S.-H., & Willis, L. A. (2007). Talking about obesity: news framing of who is responsible for causing and fixing the problem. *Journal of Health Communication, 12*(4), 359–376.

Koon, A. D., Hawkins, B., & Mayhew, S. H. (2016). Framing and the health policy process: A scoping review. *Health Policy and Planning, 31*(6), 801–816. doi:10.1093/heapol/czv128

Limb, M. (2013). Public health body quits responsibility deal over Government's failure to act on tobacco and alcohol. *British Medical Journal, 347*. doi:10.1136/bmj.f4590

Mialon, M., Swinburn, B., & Sacks, G. (2015). A proposed approach to systematically identify and monitor the corporate political activity of the food industry with respect to public health using publicly available information. *Obesity Reviews, 16*(7), 519–530.

Miller, D., & Harkins, C. (2010). Corporate strategy, corporate capture: Food and alcohol industry lobbying and public health. *Critical Social Policy, 30*(4), 564–589.

Miller, P.G., de Groot, F., McKenzie, S., & Droste, N. (2011). Vested interests in addiction research and policy. Alcohol industry use of social aspect public relations organizations against preventative health measures. *Addiction, 106*(9), 1560–1567. doi:10.1111/j.1360-0443.2011.03499.x

Moodie, R., Stuckler, D., Monteiro, C., Sheron, N., Neal, B., Thamarangsi, T., … Casswell, S. (2013). Profits and pandemics: Prevention of harmful effects of tobacco, alcohol, and ultra-processed food and drink industries. *The Lancet, 381*(9867), 670–679. doi:10.1016/S0140-6736(12)62089-3

Morrell, B., Forsyth, R., Lipworth, W., Kerridge, I., & Jordens, C. F. (2015). Rules of engagement: Journalists' attitudes to industry influence in health news reporting. *Journalism: Theory, Practice & Criticism, 16*(5), 596–614.

Nixon, L., Mejia, P., Cheyne, A., Wilking, C., Dorfman, L., & Daynard, R. (2015). "We're part of the solution": Evolution of the food and beverage industry's framing of obesity concerns between 2000 and 2012. *American Journal of Public Health, 105*(11), 2228–2236.

Panjwani, C., & Caraher, M. (2014). The Public Health Responsibility Deal: Brokering a deal for public health, but on whose terms? *Health Policy, 114*(2–3), 163–173.

Petticrew, M., Katikireddi, S. V., Knai, C., Cassidy, R., Hessari, N. M., Thomas, J., & Weishaar, H. (2017). 'Nothing can be done until everything is done': The use of complexity arguments by food, beverage, alcohol and gambling industries. *Journal of Epidemiology and Community Health, 71*(11), 1078–1083.

Picard, R. G., & Yeo, M. (2011). *Medical and health news and information in the UK media: The current state of knowledge.* University of Oxford: Reuters Institute for the Study of Journalism.

Savell, E., Fooks, G., & Gilmore, A. B. (2016). How does the alcohol industry attempt to influence marketing regulations? A systematic review. *Addiction, 111*(1), 18–32.

Snow, D. A., & Benford, R. D. (1988). Ideology, frame resonance, and participant mobilization. *International Social Movement Research, 1*(1), 197–217.

Wallack, L. (1992). Warning: The alcohol industry is not your friend? *Addiction, 87*(8), 1109–1111. doi:10.1111/j.1360-0443.1992.tb01997.x

Weiss, J. A. (1989). The powers of problem definition: The case of government paperwork. *Policy Sciences, 22*(2), 97–121.

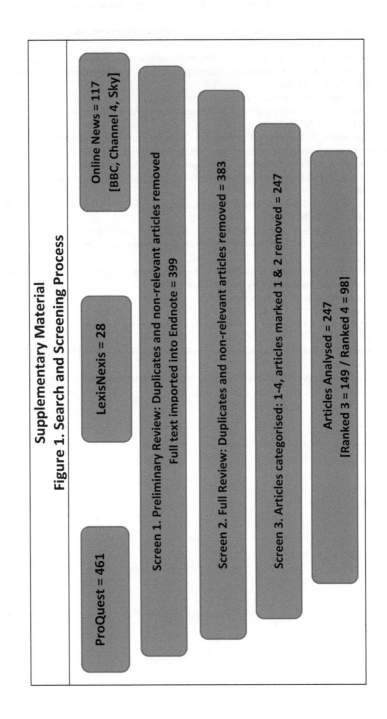

Supplementary Material
Figure 1. Search and Screening Process

ProQuest = 461

LexisNexis = 28

Online News = 117
[BBC, Channel 4, Sky]

Screen 1. Preliminary Review: Duplicates and non-relevant articles removed
Full text imported into Endnote = 399

Screen 2. Full Review: Duplicates and non-relevant articles removed = 383

Screen 3. Articles categorised: 1-4, articles marked 1 & 2 removed = 247

Articles Analysed = 247
[Ranked 3 = 149 / Ranked 4 = 98]

2 Public engagement and the role of the media in post-marketing drug safety

The case of Eltroxin® (levothyroxine) in New Zealand

Kevin Dew, John Gardner (iD), Elaine H. Morrato, Pauline Norris (iD), Kerry Chamberlain (iD), Darrin Hodgetts and Jonathan Gabe

ABSTRACT

The potential for harms from adverse drug reactions (ADR) constitutes wawcritical patient safety and public health challenge, especially with increased medication usage as populations age. The research reported here explores explanations for a sudden increase in ADR reporting in New Zealand after a new formulation of a medication to treat hypothyroidism, Eltroxin® (levothyroxine), was phased in. The formulation was adjudged to be bioequivalent to the old formulation, yet following its introduction, a sharp increase in the reporting of adverse reactions to this drug occurred. The paper analyses public engagement and the role of print media coverage, press releases and minutes of meetings of relevant agencies in order to describe the unfolding of this health controversy. Early interpretations of the sharp increase in reporting of reactions explained it as an outcome of a combination of factors, including a mistrust of state drug subsidising agencies and media attention that provoked anxiety in this vulnerable population. This paper offers an alternative explanation arguing that, as adverse drug reactions are known to be significantly underreported, the Eltroxin® 'health scare' illustrates enhanced pharmacovigilance triggered by the interaction between patients and the media. The Eltroxin® controversy is an illustrative case example of the amplification of ADR reporting by patients following increased media attention in the context of a low consumer reporting environment. The case of Eltroxin® indicates that drug safety can be enhanced by actively using media sources and by encouraging patient engagement and reporting of ADRs.

Introduction

Adverse Drug Reactions (ADRs) constitute an important public health problem in terms of mortality, morbidity and cost (Lopez-Gonzalez, Herdeiro, & Figueiras, 2009). Fatal ADRs may be as high as the fourth leading cause of death and between 1998 and 2005 reports of serious ADRs in the US increased 2.7-fold (Lazarou, Pomeranz, & Corey, 1998; Wiktorowicz, Lexchin, & Moscou, 2012). ADR surveillance, including reporting, monitoring and responding to ADRs, is a public health priority (Gibbons et al., 2010). Pharmacovigilance, a crucial element of drug safety, is the specialised surveillance activity of 'analysing and managing the risk posed by medications once they have come on to the market' (Lopez-Gonzalez et al., 2009). As a result of increasing concern over the detection of adverse drug events, pharmacovigilance systems have become more common in nation states since the 1990s (Basch, 2013; Lopez-Gonzalez et al., 2009). The World Health Organisation Uppsala Monitoring Centre, which collects and assesses information from the pharmacovigilance systems of WHO member countries, contains over three million reports of suspected adverse drug reactions (World Health Organization, 2006).

There is significant underreporting of ADRs. One systematic review suggests that underreporting rates for ADRs could be as high as 94% (Hazell & Shakir, 2006). Post-marketing underreporting of ADRs may occur as a result of hesitancy on the part of health professionals and patients to report reactions. Even with reporting systems for ADRs in place, their efficacy may be limited. For example, the United Kingdom has an online system for patients to report suspected ADRs, the Yellow Card Scheme. The Yellow Card Scheme was established in 1964 to allow health care professionals to spontaneously report adverse drug reactions to the Medicines and Healthcare Products Regulatory Agency. In 2005, the Scheme was expanded to allow patient reporting of adverse drug reactions (Avery et al., 2011). Medawar and colleagues suggest that when only health professionals could report ADRs using this Scheme patient concerns were underreported, even for medications known to have side effects or where medications have been the source of controversy, such as with particular Selective Serotonin Reuptake Inhibitor (SSRI) antidepressant medications (Medawar, Herxheimer, Bell, & Jofre, 2002). The Yellow Card system in UK hospitals was found to be used in only 6.3% of ADR cases (Smith et al., 1996).

Suspected ADRs are a frequent reason for doctor–patient contact (Miller, Britt, Valenti, & Knox, 2006); however, practitioners appear to start from the normative position that drugs released to the market are safe, and that adverse reactions reported to them can be dismissed as unreliable or a symptom of patient hypervigilance. In relation to SSRIs, Medawar and colleagues note that patients claim that doctors either deny their reports of symptoms (in this case from withdrawal of the medication) or attribute their symptoms to some other cause. These authors suggest that 'until some form of patient reporting becomes the norm, the so far unidentified but in principle avoidable harm that patients suffer from medicines will continue' (Medawar et al., 2002, p. 168). Informing patients about side effects has been described as dilemmatic in that patients have a right to being so informed but a possible consequence is that this information could deter patients from accessing beneficial treatment (Williams & Donaghue, 2010).

Many countries have made efforts to enhance public engagement in drug safety by introducing spontaneous patient reporting systems. In an 11-country survey of extant systems the level of patient reporting was variable, ranging from 1 to 2% of all reports received in New Zealand to 57% in the USA (van Hunsel, Harmark, Pal, Olsson, & van Grootheest, 2012). Patient reporting was valued for signal detection purposes, but awareness of these reporting systems amongst the general population was thought to be low. A noteworthy finding was the 6-fold increase in the number of reports submitted by consumers between 2000 and 2009 in the US co-incident with efforts to increase awareness and ease of patient reporting mechanisms.

In a systematic review of questionnaire-based research with health professionals, a number of factors that potentially inhibit reporting of ADRs were identified. Health professionals were not always aware of the kinds of reactions that need reporting and were concerned about reporting only suspected ADRs, with some holding the view that only safe drugs are released onto the market (Lopez-Gonzalez et al., 2009). Similar factors were identified in research undertaken in Sweden with general practitioners and hospital physicians. Reluctance amongst these professionals to report reactions were attributed to a lack of time and the prioritising of concerns considered more important, a lack of knowledge of existing rules, uncertainty over whether an adverse reaction was well-known or not, and hesitation to report solely on suspicion of an adverse reaction (Backstrom, Mjorndal, Dahlqvist, & Nordkvist-Olsson, 2000). Abraham (2003) argues that even when reports are made they are difficult to interpret as the quality of the data may be poor. On the patient side, it has been found that patients on anti-depressant medication experience ADRs but under-recognise them. Higher levels of under-recognition occurred in patients for whom the medication was less successful in controlling the depression (Kikuchi, Suzuki, Uchida, Watanabe, & Kashima, 2011). Physicians then underestimate ADRs and patients under-recognise them.

A few qualitative studies have explored the issue of ADRs in the consultation. An interview-based study found that most patients attending general practice consultations expressed their aversion to medications in a muted fashion (Britten, Stevenson, Gafaranga, Barry, & Bradley, 2004). In a Swedish study, 20 out of 33 patients reported side-effects from their current antihypertensive medication, but despite this, 'side effects' as a term was seldom used by patients or physicians (Kjellgren, Svensson, Ahlner, & Saljo, 1998). In consultations related to antipsychotic medication, it has been found that patient concerns are routinely underestimated. When presented with such concerns, the psychiatrist would commonly offer no response, change the subject or disagree with the patient's interpretation (Seale, Chaplin, Lelliot, & Quirk, 2007). In general practitioner consultations, GPs routinely downgrade concerns about side effects when prescribing and patients present any concerns about side effects in a heavily mitigated and circumspect fashion (Dew, Stubbe, Macdonald, & Dowell, 2012) Such avoidance of discussions of side effects may be due to the need of both participants in the consultation to save face and avoid potentially awkward or difficult exchanges (Goffman, 2006).

In summary, pharmacovigilance involves the epidemiologic surveillance of a variety of interrelated levels of reporting of ADRs, both through official and informal channels. These involve patients reporting to doctors, doctors reporting to pharmacovigilance systems, patients to patients, through conversations and social networking, and patients to journalists, in news media stories. In this article, we examine the role of media as a trigger to increased formal reporting of ADRs through a case study of a specific mediated episode. The context is a country that has patient-reporting mechanisms but they are infrequently used. In exploring this case, we consider how a further mode of reporting, the patient directly to the pharmacovigilance system, emerges when patients discover their right to report formally to such systems, revealing the inter-related nature of informal and formal systems of reporting and the importance of facilitating public engagement in drug safety.

Methods

We examined a controversial episode of ADR reporting that occurred in New Zealand in 2007 following the introduction of a new formulation of the levothyroxine medication, Eltroxin®, a prescription-only drug used to treat hypothyroidism. This case is unusual for the relatively large number of reports of adverse reactions that were made to the Centre for Adverse Reactions Monitoring (CARM) in response to the introduction of the new formulation. It is also interesting because despite the claims issued by the various monitoring agencies and the drug manufacturer that the new formulation was safe, patients' claims of adverse reactions prompted government agencies to supply and subsidise an alternative to Eltroxin®.

New Zealand has a public health system where approved drugs are provided under government subsidy. The agency responsible for regulating therapeutic products in New Zealand and overseeing drug safety activities is Medsafe (the New Zealand Medicines and Medical Devices Safety Authority, a business unit of the Ministry of Health), with responsibility for approving medications to be listed for subsidy resting with PHARMAC (the Pharmaceutical Management Agency). The New Zealand Pharmacovigilance Centre (NZPVC) is responsible for post-marketing surveillance of medications. CARM is part of the NZPVC, and relies on a spontaneous reporting scheme for adverse reactions. It has a database holding 80,000 reports of ADRs. The Medicines Adverse Reactions Committee (MARC) acts as an independent advisory committee to the Ministry of Health, and committee members are practising medical practitioners. MARC receives material from CARM and other sources, and acts as an advisor to Medsafe.

We sourced a range of relevant media material across the period of the controversy, from June 2008 when reports of ADRs first appeared to August 2009, when it was announced that three drugs would be subsidised which effectively ended media coverage of the issue. Newztext and Factiva databases were searched for media articles and press releases using the search term Eltroxin®, resulting in 65 documents. Sixteen press releases were identified from the institutional websites of PHARMAC, Medsafe, the Ministry of Health and political parties. Minutes from MARC meetings that reviewed Eltroxin® were obtained from the Medsafe website (http://www.medsafe.govt.nz/Profs/adverse.asp). A content analysis was performed to identify the sequence of events, the different actors involved and how these actors responded to the controversy, with the object of better understanding the reasons for the sharp increase in reported ADRs.

Findings

Media reports of adverse drug reactions

In July 2007, a new formulation of Eltroxin®, a drug used to treat hypothyroidism, was introduced into New Zealand and 70,000 people with hypothyroidism were phased onto the new formulation. This new formulation was a result of the manufacturer, GlaxoSmithKline, consolidating its manufacturing operations. Prior to the formulation change, CARM had received about one report every 2–3 years where thyroxine was the suspect agent, coming to a total of 14 reports of ADRs to thyroxine medications between 1973 and 2007. CARM received the first report of a problem attributed to the new formulation on 8 October 2007. After the formulation change occurred, reports of adverse reactions began to appear in the media. The new formulation was linked by various users to a range of adverse effects, from joint and muscle pain, weight gain and depression, to conjunctivitis, skin rash, and visual disturbances. Despite assurances from both the drug manufacturer and Medsafe that the new formulation was safe for use, reports of adverse reactions continued to accumulate.

The link between the new Eltroxin® formulation and a series of reported ADRs was first publicised in the regional paper *The Southland Times*, a year after the introduction of the new formulation. Published on 7 June 2008, the article heading read 'Changes to Thyroid Drug Formula Blamed for Sickness' (Gerken, 2008a). This disseminated concerns about the new formulation to a wider audience. Patients' accounts of adverse reactions after the switch to the new formulation were provided, and a local pharmacist was quoted as saying that GlaxoSmithKline and PHARMAC were trying to cover up the issue (Gerken, 2008a).

Four days later an article in *The Southland Times* elaborated on the alternative medication that patients claimed did not cause adverse reactions, levothyroxine manufactured by Goldshield Ltd (Southland Times, 2008). Because it was not subsidised by PHARMAC, patients had to pay the full cost of this medication themselves. Less than 40% of New Zealanders have private health insurance with very few having coverage for medication in primary care (Cumming et al., 2014). As a result PHARMAC's decisions about what to subsidise strongly determines what is accessible to patients. In another article published three days after this in *The Southland Times* the first line reads: 'The Centre for Adverse Reactions Monitoring [CARM] wants to hear from Eltroxin® users who have suffered side-effects since the thyroid treatment drug was reformulated' (Gerken, 2008e). CARM is part of the New Zealand Pharmacovigilance Centre located at the University of Otago, and instructions on how to contact the centre were provided at the end of the article. By providing these instructions to Eltroxin® users, the media opened up a channel for these users to contact CARM directly. Although direct patient reporting to CARM was already a possibility, it is unlikely that patients were aware it existed or, if they were, they may not have realised that they could make reports directly to CARM. To illustrate, there are pamphlets on adverse reactions to vaccines that could be displayed in GP waiting rooms that mention CARM, but these pamphlets state that patients should inform their GPs about any reactions and provide no information on how to access CARM directly.

After this initial coverage by *The Southland Times*, media coverage quickly spread to other parts of the country and subsequently a greater number of individuals claimed to be having adverse reactions to the new drug. On June 17 *The Waikato Times* published an article providing an account of a woman who was rushed to hospital with vision and memory loss, vomiting, diarrhoea, and crippling arthritic pain after switching to Eltroxin® (Akoorie, 2008). Her pharmacist was so shocked by her reaction that he posted a sign in his shop asking any users to alert staff if they have problems. Articles then appear in *The Otago Daily Times* on July 3, *The Timaru Herald* on July 21 and *The Nelson Mail* on July 28.

Regulatory and political actors respond to the media reports

On 27 June 2008 Medsafe issued a press release. This stated that Medsafe had reassessed the changes in Eltroxin® formulation and could confirm that it 'satisfies all quality, safety and bioequivalence criteria' and all 'excipients and excipient quantities present in the new formulation are commonly used in medicines'. Excipients are not regarded as pharmacologically active substances but bind and deliver the active ingredient of the medication. The press release then suggests that 'poor patient compliance should be considered as a possible cause of adverse effects' (Medsafe, 2008a). The August 22 edition of *The Southland Times* claimed that most people who switched to the Goldshield brand, which could be purchased at an unsubsidised price, had felt better within a couple of days (Gerken, 2008d). Jackie Blue, a Member of Parliament in opposition, entered the controversy by issuing a press release on August 22 claiming that 'MPs from all parties have been inundated with calls from constituents whose health is being seriously affected by the new formulation of Eltroxin' (Blue, 2008b). This was followed by a small burst of media activity with *The Southland Times* revisiting the controversy on 27 August (Gerken, 2008c). On 28 August, *The National Business Review* carried a headline that over 500 complaints had been made about the drug's side effects (The National Business Review, 2008). This article attracted 167 on-line comments, primarily of people reporting side effects after switching to Eltroxin®. These concerns were repeated by other politicians who joined in with their own press releases. The Green Party issued a press release on 28 August with the heading 'Situation critical for thyroid sufferers' (Kedgley, 2008). The next day articles appeared in *The Press*, a Christchurch paper, and *The Dominion Post*, a Wellington paper. Jackie Blue issued another press release on 8 September with the headline 'Action on Eltroxin now urgent', which ended with a recommendation that anyone experiencing symptoms should contact CARM (Blue, 2008a). *The National Business Review* published articles on the two days following this press release and on 10 September; questions were raised in Parliament on this issue where it was announced that the government was looking at the possibility of subsidising alternatives to Eltroxin® (Office of the Clerk, 2008).

On 11 September 2008, the Eltroxin® formulation change and adverse reactions were discussed at the Medicines Adverse Reactions Committee (MARC). This began with a discussion of a report submitted to the committee from CARM stating that before October 2007 only 14 reports of ADRs had been received for thyroxine, but since then 810 reports of suspected adverse reactions had been received. Over 40% of the reports were made by patients, a marked increase on the 1–2% of total reports to CARM typically received from patients (MARC, 2008). Usually, nearly all reports are made by general practitioners.

Table 1 presents a summary of the analysis of 576 of the reports received by CARM and fully processed between October 2007 and August 2008 (Tatley, 2008). Three types of symptoms were most commonly

Table 1. Analysis of Eltroxin® reports received by CARM (8 October 2007–31 August 2008).

	All	Hypothyroid[b]	Headache	Hyper-sensitivity	Conjunctivitis/ Eye	Acute Upper GI	Vision
Reactions, N (row %)	576 (100%)	364 (28.6%)	165 (28.6%)	161 (28.0%)	158 (27.4%)	110 (19.1%)	106 (18.4%)
Sole Medicine[a], column %	70.0	69.0	70.3	70.2	71.5	65.5	66.0
Known Onset, column %	N = 252	N = 156	N = 63	N = 70	N = 66	N = 49	N = 46
≤24 hours	14.7	10.3	15.9	14.3	15.2	32.7	6.5
≾1 week	19.0	16.7	23.8	22.9	18.2	20.4	17.4
<1 month	40.9	42.3	38.1	37.1	28.8	32.7	43.5
<3 months	13.1	18.6	9.5	15.7	19.7	6.1	13.0
>3 months	12.3	12.2	12.7	10.0	18.2	8.2	19.6

Source: The Eltroxin formulation change: An analysis of reports received by CARM (Tatley, 2008).
[a]'Sole medicine' refers to Eltroxin® being the only medication mentioned in the report.
[b]Hypothyroid symptoms include weakness, fatigue, cold intolerance, constipation, weight gain, depression, joint or muscle pain, brittle fingernails/hair, slow speech, dry skin, puffy face, hands and feet, decreased taste and smell, thinning of eyebrows, hoarseness and abnormal menstrual periods.

described: hypothyroid-type symptoms (53.2%); headache (28.6% of reports, and also associated with visual disturbances, 18.4% of reactions) and hypersensitivity (28.0%). In 7.8% of the reports, there was mention of additional lab tests to evaluate T4 and TSH hormone levels. In 70.0% of the reports, Eltroxin was the sole medication. Amongst the reports with known onset of symptoms, three quarters were reported to have occurred within a month of drug initiation. Dechallenge, where administration of the drug is stopped to observe changes in ADRs, occurred in about 90% of the reported cases and of these, 17.7% improved upon stopping but did not continue medication and 72.1% elected to continue medication. For CARM the headache, visual and additional conjunctivitis/eye problems (27.4% of reports) were of particular concern because there was no clear explanation for them (Tatley, 2008). Reports had been received from across New Zealand, although a disproportionate number were from Southland. The committee was also told that the Pharmacovigilance Centre had contacted 83 countries on the World Health Organization adverse reactions monitoring scheme. There had been no reports of adverse reactions to the new GlaxoSmithKline formulation, although similar adverse reactions had been reported in some countries to other brands of thyroxine.

MARC noted that the Medsafe Compliance Team had not found any obvious quality or manufacturing reason for the increased number of adverse reaction reports. This team also confirmed the Good Manufacturing Practice (GMP) of the product's site of manufacture, and the results of independent tests were reported to the committee. Four batches of the new Eltroxin° formulation had been tested, including a batch returned by a patient who had reported adverse reactions. No contaminants were identified. Impurities, present in both the old and new formulations, were well within accepted levels, and an assay of the active ingredient indicated that it was well within the specification (MARC, 2008). Medsafe also reported that it had consulted expert endocrinologists in June 2008 and again in August 2008. The more minor reactions could be attributed to changes in how patients ingested the medication: the old formulation pill could be broken in half, allowing for half a pill to be taken twice a day, whereas the new formulation had to be taken as one whole pill at least once a day. The endocrinologists, however, were unable to explain some of the more severe symptoms being reported, particularly visual disturbances.

After considering the reports of both CARM and Medsafe, the Committee concluded that there was no 'specific medical, physiological or pharmacological explanation for the increase in adverse reaction reports'. But it also noted that reports of improvement after switching brands added weight to the argument that there may be some link. Consequently, the committee then initiated two further actions. Firstly, it recommended that Medsafe continue to work with PHARMAC to encourage an alternative brand to be approved and supplied in New Zealand. Secondly, the committee recommended that Medsafe, in conjunction with the Pharmacovigilance Centre, continue to monitor adverse reactions reports and inform the committee of any further developments.

The Ministry of Health produced a press release on 11 September 2008, which discredited a number of claims, including that the formulation was manufactured in India and contained genetically engineered ingredients (Ministry of Health, 2008). None of these claims were apparent in any of the printed media coverage of the controversy.

Thyroxine alternatives are made accessible to patients

Many patients were turning to Goldshield as a better alternative, even though it could only be purchased at the unsubsidised price. According to an article in *The Press*, the company responsible for supplying the unsubsidised drug to New Zealand could not obtain enough supplies to keep up with demand (Wylie, 2008). Pharmacists directly imported stocks of levothryroxine (Goldshield) manufactured in the United Kingdom and Synthroid (levothyroxine, Abbott Laboratories) manufactured in Canada (Gerken, 2008b).

On the 30th of September, PHARMAC announced that it had signed a provisional agreement with the supplier of Goldshield: if Goldshield was approved for distribution by Medsafe, it would be listed in Section B of the Pharmaceutical Schedule, establishing it as a subsidised medication (PHARMAC, 2008). In a later press release from Medsafe, assurances were given that the addition of Goldshield would not result in any changes to the subsidisation of Eltroxin° (Medsafe, 2008b). Another brand, Synthroid, had also been given provisional limited consent for distribution. Use of both these products was limited to the initiation of treatment in new patients and to those patients who were intolerant to the other brands. The press release also confirmed that this would mean that Goldshield would be fully subsidised alongside Eltroxin®, and that PHARMAC had been making arrangements to ensure large stocks of the new subsidised drug would be available from November onwards (Medsafe, 2008b). After the introduction of the new subsidised Goldshield, media coverage quickly became much less frequent, as did reporting of ADRs.

Table 2 outlines the relationship between the reporting of ADRs and media coverage. From this history of events it can be seen that the media produced a particular rendering of Eltroxin®, with only one article in *The National Business Review* presenting the view of the drug manufacturer (Hall, 2008). In addition, the print media publicised the existence of CARM and the means by which to contact CARM and formally report concerns. This media activity was consolidated by the actions of politicians issuing press releases, which again publicised CARM but in addition provided material for further press coverage.

Discussion

This paper has described the timeline of events that concerned a more than 400-fold increase in patient-reported ADRs for Eltroxin® in New Zealand. Several mechanisms have been proposed to understand the increased ADR reporting rate observed with Eltroxin®: (1) biomedical; (2) human factors; and (3) systemic changes in drug safety reporting.

Changes in product formulation as explanation for increased ADR reporting

The reports of ADRs were a puzzle to the regulatory public health agencies concerned with drug safety. First of all, the type and quantity of the active ingredient, levothyroxine (also commonly referred to as thyroxine), was unchanged. It was only the non-active ingredients, the excipients, that were changed, and the excipients in the new formulation were very common and widely used in other medications.

The new formulation was adjudged to be the bioequivalent of the old formulation. The Medsafe website states that 'Bioequivalence is determined by comparing as a ratio, the rate and extent of absorption, metabolism and excretion (plasma profile) of two medicines in the body' (Medsafe, 2010). With the new formulation, the information provided by GlaxoSmithKline showed that bioequivalence fell within an internationally accepted range of 0.8–1.25. The issue of bioequivalence between branded and generic levothyroxine has been contested in the USA. In a joint statement the American Thyroid Association, The Endocrine Society, and American Association of Clinical Endocrinologists argue that 'levothyroxine is a drug recognized to have a narrow toxic to therapeutic ratio with significant clinical consequences of excessive or inadequate treatment' (American Thyroid Association, The Endocrine Society, & American Association of Clinical Endocrinologists, 2004). So although the view in New Zealand was that the new formulation of Eltroxin® was bioequivalent, the 80–125% range of bioequivalence is broad compared to the narrow toxic to therapeutic ratio of the medication. A survey of American physicians prescribing thyroxine found that switching between approved preparations continued to be associated with some adverse outcomes, frequently resulting from generic substitution without the prescriber's knowledge (Hennessey, Malabanan, Haugen, & Levy, 2010). Switching between thyroxine-containing products can usually be managed by re-adjusting the dosage. However, for CARM this may lead to a short-term increase in reported ADRs during the phase of dose titration.

Human factors as explanation for increased ADR reporting

It has been argued that the Eltroxin® episode resulted from an irrational response from hypothyroid patients, where media coverage, distrust of PHARMAC and the agitation of a few key individuals encouraged a group of patients prone to emotional distress to attribute their various health problems to the

Table 2. Eltroxin® coverage and ADR reports.

Unfolding of events	Key message in media reports	Official ADR reports
		CARM database records 14 events since 1965
July 2007 – new formulation		
7 June 2008 – First article appears in *Southland Times*	Report from patient with side effects she blamed on the base ingredients. Local pharmacist suggests a cover-up	8 Oct 2007 – First report of ADR from Eltroxin®
14 June 2008 – *Southland Times* publishes article with CARM contact information	CARM director says if reports of ADRs are true people should contact CARM	
17 June 2008 – *Waikato Times* article	Report of women admitted to hospital after taking new formulation	
27 2008 – MedSafe press release	Confirms that Eltroxin® meets all quality and bioequivalence criteria	
3 July 2008 – *Otago Daily Times* article	200 ADRs reported	
21 July 2008 – *Timaru Herald* article	350 ADRs reported but patients had to pay for an alternative	
28 July 2008– *Nelson Mail* article	Describes symptoms from alleged 400 reports received by CARM	
22 August 2008 – *Southland Times*	Reports on patients demands to subsidise Goldshield as an alternative	
27 August 2008 – *Southland Times* article	Reports on new patient website and 600 ADRs	
28 August 2008 – *National Business Review* article	Reports that Government is seeking an additional supplier	
		2 Sept 2008 – 746 ADRs reported (1% of pts)
		11 Sept 2008 – 810 ADRs reported
30 Sept 2008 – PHARMAC subsidises Goldshield		

new drug formulation, evidenced by reporting of ADRs increasing after television coverage (Faasse, Cundy, & Petrie, 2010; Faasse, Gamble, Cundy, & Petrie, 2012). This explanation for the patient report-ing of ADRs is premised on the normative position that the new formulation was, in fact, safe for use and equivalent to the old version. The high number of ADRs could therefore be explained away as an *over*-reporting of adverse reactions by *irrational* patients. While this argument may have some poten-tial relevance for the episode, it both underestimates the rationality of patients and oversimplifies the complex, socially mediated role of media in health communication and the important place of public engagement in drug safety. This type of account is not uncommon. There has been a tradition of dis-missing patient reports of safety problems with medicines which has thus further exposed people to unsafe products (Abraham & Shepherd, 1999; Mintz, 1985).

Changes in drug safety reporting mechanisms as explanation for increased ADR reporting

The way that the Eltroxin® 'health scare' played out in news coverage facilitated a particular process of reporting ADRs that is missing under the usual institutionalised arrangements for ADR reporting in New Zealand. Over the course of the controversy, the customary channels for ADR reporting were augmented, and a novel pharmacovigilance arrangement emerged. From this perspective, the Eltroxin® controversy did not constitute an over-reporting of adverse reactions, but rather allowed for an enhanced level of reporting and registering of patient concerns. The mass media is well known for playing an important part in disseminating information in relation to health scares (Hooker, 2010). The mass media enables and prompts the public to become engaged when health concerns are raised and media coverage can influence other agencies to act. Gabe and Bury (1996), for example, argue that medication regulating agencies in the UK suspended the licence for the drug Halcion® (triazolam, Upjohn) partly in response to media coverage about the negative side effects of the drug (Gabe & Bury, 1996). The mass media provide a platform for experts and patients to mobilise public opinion.

The usual and Eltroxin® ADR reporting mechanisms are graphically illustrated in Figure 1.

Under the usual surveillance process, GPs and other health professionals are the typical source of ADR reports in New Zealand. However, there are several barriers to reporting with this mechanism. First, the patient has to consider his or her symptom to be a result of the prescribed medication. This could be particularly difficult, especially with people with co-morbidities or chronic illness that has some fluctuation in symptoms. Second, the patient has to confront the health professional, usually the one who prescribed the medication in the case of the general practitioner, with the bad news that a prescribed medication is causing problems. This is a face-threatening act in that it threatens the face of the health professional because something they have done with good intentions has caused harm (Goffman, 2006). Patients may be reluctant to engage in such face-threatening acts (Dew et al., 2012). Third, research suggests that health professionals consistently dismiss patient claims that a prescribed drug is the cause of symptoms (Backstrom et al., 2000; Lopez-Gonzalez et al., 2009; Medawar et al., 2002; Seale et al., 2007; Smith et al., 1996).

The augmented Eltroxin® process of ADR reporting is shown on the right side of Figure 1. With media involvement, patients who read or hear media reports can now potentially relate their symp-toms to the medication they are taking. This may help overcome the first barrier. GPs and other health professionals may, due to the media coverage, become more aware of the possibility that symptoms the patient presents with are a result of a medication. Politicians can be alerted by patients directly or through media coverage and in turn facilitate further coverage. Cumulatively, these processes can have at least two consequences: Firstly, GPs may be more likely to take a patient's association of symptoms with the medication as a real possibility; and secondly, GPs may themselves make the connection between a patient's symptoms and their medication without the patient making that connection. This provides more opportunities for associations to be made and ADRs to be reported. We can still anticipate underreporting here. Even if patients associate symptoms with the medication they may not wish to threaten the face of the health professional. However, with the media providing details about who to report ADRs to, patients can go directly to CARM and by-pass the health professional, thus avoiding the

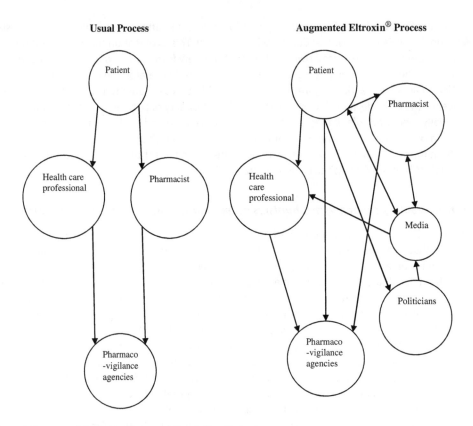

Figure 1. Processes of alerting to adverse reactions in New Zealand.

face-threatening act. This is precisely how it occurred in the Eltroxin® controversy, with CARM receiving an unusually high number of reports directly from patients. Although it was always possible for patients to report ADRs directly to CARM, they were unaware of this opportunity and it has not previously been utilised. It is, then, little wonder that there were higher rates of ADR reports where media coverage of the controversy was extensive.

The importance of different means of ascertaining ADRs is highlighted by Hennessey and colleagues' pharmacovigilance survey of practitioners regarding the safety of substitution of L-thyroxine products. They found that a survey of practitioners generated 5-fold more cases of adverse drug experience reports than received over a seven-year period by the FDA (Hennessey et al., 2010).

The role of PHARMAC is undoubtedly important in the playing out of this controversy as well. As it initially subsidised only Eltroxin® and not other medications it was less likely that those patients would switch to other medications to treat hypothyroidism – as they would have to pay the full, unsubsidised cost and supplies of such drugs were limited. This meant that media could only describe the problems, and not offer solutions to patients except the possibility of paying for the unsubsidised medications if they were available at local pharmacies. In other countries where the new formulation was introduced, Germany and the Netherlands, alternative brands were available and no significant increases in ADRs occurred (MARC, 2008). In effect, this meant there was no 'release valve' to divert concerns about ADRs in New Zealand as there was in other jurisdictions where the new formula was used.

Implications for drug safety and public health practices

From this study of Eltroxin®, it can be concluded that the customary surveillance channels for ADR reporting were augmented and a more dynamic pharmacovigilance arrangement emerged as a result of public engagement. Active pharmacovigilance surveillance systems, such as occur in the USA, are reliant on patient recording to detect post-marketing concerns about ADRs as part of a multi-prong strategy that includes government-sponsored networks of population databases, use of data mining approaches and formal integration of these diverse sources of drug safety information (Hennessey et al., 2010; Smith & Benattia, 2016; Wiktorowicz et al., 2012). In the Netherlands a website for patient reporting has been in place since 2003 and in the UK online patient reporting has been available since 2005 (Avery et al., 2011). New Zealand's Intensive Medicines Monitoring Programme has trialled enhanced patient involvement in reporting in relation to one medication, Dapoxetine (Priligy®). This trial included a request to doctors to pass on reporting forms to patients (Harrison-Woolrych, 2011). The results of this trial have not been released and in 2013 the Intensive Medicines Monitoring Programme closed. Efforts to incorporate patient perspectives are in response to current reporting being heavily reliant on reporting from health care professionals and evidence that suggests that improvements in the accuracy of ADR data can be achieved by collecting data directly from patients (Banerjee et al., 2013). Patient reporting provides more detailed descriptions of ADRs, their impact on daily life, and reports are obtained on different drugs when compared to health-care professional reporting (Avery et al., 2011; Inácio, Cavaco, & Airaksinen, 2016).

The analysis here suggests other possible means to enhance ADR reporting by patients after approval of pharmaceuticals that Banerjee et al. classify as an approach where patient selection is not restrictive and the population from which reporting is obtained is not prespecified (Banerjee et al., 2013). Firstly, patient information exchange could be developed so that patients on medications are able to recognise their symptoms as possible ADRs. Medawar and colleagues argue that Internet sites, which act as patient support groups, allowing patients to tell their medication stories, can act in this way (Medawar et al., 2002). Saukko (Saukko, 2009) provides an example of this in relation to a thrombophilia online group, where participants could consider whether or not their symptoms were related to anticoagulant medication when others made these claims. By reading the stories of others, patients can consider the validity of their own stories. Secondly, patients should be made aware of such sites. Public health agencies who regulate prescription medicines could house these sites, and when a patient is prescribed a new medication, information could be provided to patients on how to access them. Pharmacists have been described as being 'uncomfortable with persuading patients to take fewer medications' (Jesson & Bissell, 2006, p. 168) but could play an important role in positioning themselves as potential recipients of patient concerns about side effects. Thirdly, these stories need to be heard by regulators and drug manufacturers who are responsible for drug safety surveillance. This can be achieved in at least two ways. The first enhanced approach uses a passive strategy, where patients are provided with information on how to report an ADR officially. The drug safety agencies can then passively receive these reports. For example, in the United States, the Food and Drug Administration Amendments Act (FDAAA) of 2007 mandated that printed direct-to-consumer advertisements for prescription drugs include the following statement presented in conspicuous text: 'You are encouraged to report negative side effects of prescription drugs to the FDA. Visit www.fda.gov/medwatch, or call 1-800-FDA-1088'. The MedWatch Safety Information and Adverse Event Reporting Program is a voluntary reporting system in which manufacturers, health care providers and patients can submit adverse event reports via phone, fax or Internet. Reporting information is also provided in patient medication guides and FDA drug safety alerts.

The second enhanced approach uses an active strategy, where the public health agencies who regulate prescriptions medicines enhance the scope of their surveillance by conducting systematic analyses of patient websites to identify possible ADR signals and their possible impacts. This aligns with Medawar and colleagues view that agencies should immerse themselves in the stories told by medication users (Medawar et al., 2002), and Banerjee et al's discussion of the examination of free text from social web sites (Banerjee et al., 2013). Research on a specifically formed ADR Facebook page found that such a forum produced a high yield of reported ADRs (Knezevic, Bivolarevic, Peric, & Jankovic, 2011). The suggestion here is that similar research could be undertaken in relation to specific conditions (such as hypothyroidism) to identify the utility of social media in identifying ADRs. On the other hand, monitoring of social media for mentions of adverse reactions, as is required by a European

Union directive has been shown to identify ADR reports at a similar volume to existing adverse event reporting channels (Edwards & Lindquist, 2011; Kmetz, 2011) That is, where all social media sites are data mined the conclusions may be little different from standard reporting, but monitoring sites that have been set up specifically to explore the topic of ADRs or of a particular condition may provide more reports. Multi-prong approaches in surveillance need to synthesise evidence from a range of sources to provide a more complete picture of drug risk.

Media provides another channel for promoting enhanced ADR reporting. However, we do not seek to promote media-centricism, where the media are positioned as producing the primary causal effect (Silverstone, 2007). Rather, we consider news media to be part of existing ADR reporting processes at both formal and informal levels. It is well established that media pervade contemporary society and processes of health communication (Hodgetts & Chamberlain, 2006; Silverstone, 1999). Stories circulated through news media can establish other opportunities for reporting, such as the establishment of patient support groups and websites, and they can facilitate discussions of ADRs in patient–doctor interactions. For example, Medawar and colleagues note that television publicity associated with Seroxat® (paroxetine) contributed to many user reports about the drug effects being posted on websites. Many users stated that prior to seeing the comments of others on these websites, they had not associated their symptoms with the medications in question (Medawar et al., 2002). In the case of Eltroxin®, support groups and websites were established and, in addition, regional newspapers played an important role in disseminating information. There is potential here for drug safety agencies to make more use of smaller regional newspapers, often more eager to have news stories, to publicise concerns and raise their own profiles. Taken together, these processes suggest that there can be considerable benefit from utilising diverse public engagement processes to enhance the reporting of ADRs and consequently improve drug safety surveillance, achieving a public health goal of minimising the effects of preventable adverse reactions to drugs.

Conclusions

It has been argued in this paper that dismissing aberrant responses of adverse reactions to medications as an outcome of a health scare is inadequate. There is strong evidence that ADRs continue to be significantly under-reported. As such, it is imperative that drug safety agencies and pharmacovigilance managers continue to respond to the important public health issue of ADRs and to the problem of their under-reporting. Health researchers and policy-makers should take care in concluding that certain players in a drug safety controversy are irrational whilst others are rational. Careful attention needs to be paid to the institutional means by which patient drug safety concerns are elicited if we are to tackle the problems associated with ADRs seriously. The Eltroxin® case illustrates how media coverage may have augmented the reporting of suspected adverse drug reactions by patients and health providers. Therefore, we recommend that drug safety agencies and pharmacovigilance managers should be tracking major media coverage as well as spontaneous reports in order to interpret changes in post-marketing ADR reporting rates appropriately. They should also make use of the media to raise concerns and disseminate useful information. Finally, they should also consider novel forms of accessing patient stories and facilitating public engagement, such as the use of specific social media fora, in order to identify potential pharmaceutical post-marketing concerns.

Acknowledgement

We would like to thank Michael Tatley of the Centre for Adverse Reactions Monitoring for initial discussions and information provided about the case.

Disclosure statement

No potential conflict of interest was reported by the authors.

Funding

This work was supported by the Health Research Council of New Zealand [grant number 08/256]; Dr. Morrato's contribution was supported by [grant number K12HS019464] from the Agency for Healthcare Research and Quality. The content is solely the responsibility of the authors and does not necessarily represent the official views of the Agency for Healthcare Research and Quality.

ORCID

John Gardner ⓘ http://orcid.org/0000-0001-7417-348X
Pauline Norris ⓘ http://orcid.org/0000-0003-1656-871X
Kerry Chamberlain ⓘ http://orcid.org/0000-0002-1011-4293

References

Abraham, J. (2003). Learning from drug disasters and reforming medicines regulation. *Critical Public Health, 13*, 269–279.

Abraham, J., & Shepherd, J. (1999). *The therapeutic nightmare: The battle over the world's most controversial sleeping pill.* Abingdon: Earthscan.

Akoorie, N. (2008, June 17). Woman blames drug for illness. *Waikato Times.*

American Thyroid Association, The Endocrine Society, & American Association of Clinical Endocrinologists. (2004). Joint Statement on the U.S. Food and Drug Administration's Decision Regarding Bioequivalence of Levothyroxine Sodium. Retrieved from http://www.endo-society.org/advocacy/legislative/upload/Joint_Statement_Levothyroxine-Thyroxine.pdf

Avery, A., Anderson, C., Bond, C., Fortnum, H., Gifford, A., Hannaford, P., Hazell, L., et al. (2011). Evaluation of patient reporting of adverse drug reactions to the UK 'Yellow Card Scheme': Literature review, descriptive and qualitative analyses, and questionnaire surveys. *Health Technology Assessment, 15*, 1–234. doi:10.3310/hta15200

Backstrom, M., Mjorndal, T., Dahlqvist, R., & Nordkvist-Olsson, T. (2000). Attitudes to reporting adverse drug reactions in northern Sweden. *European Journal of Clinical Pharmacology, 56*, 729–732.

Banerjee, A., Okun, S., Edwards, I. R., Wicks, P., Smith, M., Mayall, S., … Basch, E. (2013). Patient-reported outcome measures in safety event reporting: PROSPER Consortium guidance. *Drug Safety, 36*, 1129–1149.

Basch, E. (2013). New frontiers in patient-reported outcomes: Adverse event reporting, comparative effectiveness, and quality assessment. *Annual Review of Medicine, 65*, 307–317.

Blue, J. (2008a, September 8). *Press release: Action on Eltroxin now urgent.* Wellington: The National Party.

Blue, J. (2008b, August 22). *Press release: Thyroxine concerns need sorting out.* Wellington: The National Party.

Britten, N., Stevenson, F., Gafaranga, J., Barry, C., & Bradley, C. (2004). The expression of aversion to medicines in general practice consultations. *Social Science & Medicine, 59*, 1495–1503.

Cumming, J., McDonald, J., Barr, C., Martin, G., Gerring, Z., & Daubé, J. (2014). New Zealand health system review. *Health Systems in Transition, 4*, 1–242.

Dew, K., Stubbe, M., Macdonald, L., & Dowell, A. (2012). Side effects talk in general practice consultations. In B. Bates & R. Ahmed (Eds.), *Medical communication in clinical contexts* (pp. 95–126). Dubuque, IA: Kendall Hunt.

Edwards, I. R., & Lindquist, M. (2011). Social media and networks in pharmacovigilance boon or bane? *Drug Safety, 34*, 267–271.

Faasse, K., Cundy, T., & Petrie, K. (2010). Thyroxine: Anatomy of a health scare. *British Medical Journal, 340*, 20–21.

Faasse, K., Gamble, G., Cundy, T., & Petrie, K. (2012). Impact of television coverage on the number and type of symptoms reported during a health scare: A retrospective pre-post observational study. *British Medical Journal Open, 2*, e001607.

Gabe, J., & Bury, M. (1996). Halcion nights: A sociological account of a medical controversy. *Sociology, 30*, 447–469.

Gerken, S. (2008a, June 7). Changes to thyroid drug formula blamed for sickness. *The Southland Times.*

Gerken, S. (2008b, September 23). Huge demand for alternative drug. *The Southland Times.*

Gerken, S. (2008c, August 27). NZ too small for drug says Ministry. *The Southland Times.*

Gerken, S. (2008d, August 22). Patient seek new safer pills. *The Southland Times.*

Gerken, S. (2008e, June 14). Thyroid drug users urged to contact centre. *The Southland Times.*

Gibbons, R. D., Amatya, A. K., Brown, C. H., Hur, K., Marcus, S. M., Bhaumik, D. K., & Mann, J. J. (2010). Post-approval drug safety surveillance. *Annual Review of Public Health, 31*, 419–437. doi:10.1146/annurev.publhealth.012809.103649

Goffman, E. (2006). On face-work. In G. Massey (Ed.), *Readings for sociology* (pp. 105–114). New York, NY: W.W. Norton and Company.

Hall, M. (2008, September 9). The Eltroxin controversy: GlaxoSmithKline responds. *The National Business Review.*

Harrison-Woolrych, M. (2011). Patient reporting encouraged during monitoring of Dapoxetine in New Zealand. *Drug Safety, 34*, 1115–1116.

Hazell, L., & Shakir, S. A. W. (2006). Under-reporting of adverse drug reactions – A systematic review. *Drug Safety, 29*, 385–396.

Hennessey, J., Malabanan, A., Haugen, B., & Levy, E. (2010, February). Adverse event reporting in patients treated with Levothyroxine: Results of the Pharmacovigilance Task Force survey of the American Thyroid Association, American Association of of Clinical Endocrinologists and The Endocrine Society. *Endocrine Practice, 11*, 1–41.

Hodgetts, D., & Chamberlain, K. (2006). An extended media research agenda for health psychology. *Journal of Health Psychology, 11*, 317–327.

Hooker, C. (2010). Health scares: Professional priorities. *Health, 14*, 3–21. doi:10.1177/1363459309341875

van Hunsel, F., Harmark, L., Pal, S., Olsson, S., & van Grootheest, K. (2012). Experiences with adverse drug reaction reporting by patients an 11-country survey. *Drug Safety, 35*, 45–60.

Inácio, P., Cavaco, A., & Airaksinen, M. (2016). The value of patient reporting to the pharmacovigilance system: A systematic review. *British Journal of Clinical Pharmacology, 83*, 227–246. doi:10.1111/bcp.13098

Jesson, J., & Bissell, P. (2006). Public health and pharmacy: A critical review. *Critical Public Health, 16*, 159–169.

Kedgley, S. (2008, August 28). *Press release: Situation critical for thyroid sufferers: Greens*. The Green Party.

Kikuchi, T., Suzuki, T., Uchida, H., Watanabe, K., & Kashima, H. (2011). Subjective recognition of adverse events with antidepressant in people with depression: A prospective study. *Journal of Affective Disorders, 135*, 347–353.

Kjellgren, K. I., Svensson, S., Ahlner, J., & Saljo, R. (1998). Antihypertensive medication in clinical encounters. *International Journal of Cardiology, 64*, 161–169.

Kmetz, J. (2011). *Adverse event reporting in social media*. Bellevue, WA: Visible Technologies.

Knezevic, M., Bivolarevic, I., Peric, T., & Jankovic, S. (2011). Using facebook to increase spontaneous reporting of adverse drug reactions. *Drug Safety, 34*, 351–352.

Lazarou, J., Pomeranz, B. H., & Corey, P. N. (1998). Incidence of adverse drug reactions in hospitalized patients: A meta-analysis of prospective studies. *Journal of the American Medical Association, 279*, 1200–1205.

Lopez-Gonzalez, E., Herdeiro, M. T., & Figueiras, A. (2009). Determinants of under-reporting of adverse drug reactions: A systematic review. *Drug Safety, 32*, 19–31.

MARC. (2008). *Minutes of 135th Meeting held on 11 September 2008*. Wellington: Medicines Adverse Reactions Monitoring Committee.

Medawar, C., Herxheimer, A., Bell, A., & Jofre, S. (2002). Paroxetine, Panorama and user reporting of ADRs: Consumer intelligence matters in clinical practice and post-marketing drug surveillance. *International Journal of Risk & Safety in Medicine, 15*, 161–169.

Medsafe. (2008a, June 27). Press release: Eltroxin formulation change. *Scoop media limited*.

Medsafe. (2008b, October 23). Press release: Medsafe approves additional Levothyroxine products. *Scoop media limited*.

Medsafe. (2010). Eltroxin formulation change. Retrieved September 3, 2010, from http://www.medsafe.govt.nz/hot/alerts/EltroxinInfo.asp

Miller, G. C., Britt, H. C., Valenti, L., & Knox, S. (2006). Adverse drug events: Counting is not enough, action is needed [Comment]. *Medical Journal of Australia, 184*, 19.

Ministry of Health. (2008, September 11). *Media Research: Eltroxin*. Wellington: Ministry of Heatlh.

Mintz, M. (1985). *At any cost: Corporate greed, women, and the Dalkon Shield*. New York, NY: Pantheon Books.

Office of the Clerk. (2008, September 10). Press release: Questions and Answers: Wednesday. *Scoop media limited*. Retrieved from http://www.scoop.co.nz/stories/PA0809/S00234.htm

PHARMAC. (2008, September 30). Press release: Consultation on alternative thyroid treatment. *Scoop media limited*.

Saukko, P. (2009). Genetic risk online and offline: Two ways of being susceptible to blood clots. *Health, Risk and Society, 11*(1), 1–16.

Seale, C., Chaplin, R., Lelliot, P., & Quirk, A. (2007). Antipsychotic medication, sedation and mental clouding: An observational study of psychiatric consultations. *Social Science & Medicine, 65*, 698–711.

Silverstone, R. (1999). *Why study the media?* London: Sage.

Silverstone, R. (2007). *Media and morality: On the rise of the mediapolis*. Cambridge: Polity.

Smith, M., & Benattia, I. (2016). The patient's voice in pharmacovigilance: Pragmatic approaches to builing a patient-centric drug safety organization. *Drug Safety, 39*, 779–785. doi:10.1007/s40264-016-0426-9

Smith, C. C., Bennett, P. M., Pearce, H. M., Harrison, P. I., Reynolds, D. J. M., Aronson, J. K., & GrahameSmith, D. G. (1996). Adverse drug reactions in a hospital general medical unit meriting notification to the Committee on Safety of Medicines. *British Journal of Clinical Pharmacology, 42*, 423–429.

Southland Times. (2008, June 11). Hundreds more claim thyroid drug side effects. *Southland Times*.

Tatley, M. (2008). *The Eltroxin formulation change: An analysis of reports received by CARM*. Dunedin: New Zealand Pharmacovigilance Centre.

The National Business Review. (2008, August 28). Over 500 complain of side effects from drug. *The National Business Review*.

Wiktorowicz, M., Lexchin, J., & Moscou, K. (2012). Pharmacovigilance in Europe and North America: Divergent approaches. *Social Science & Medicine, 75*, 165–170.

Williams, A., & Donaghue, N. (2010). 'Now that's a fair dinkum academic debate, but this affects people's lives': A discursive analysis of arguments for and against the provision of warnings about potential side effects of SSRIs in a public debate. *Critical Public Health, 20*, 15–24.

World Health Organization (2006). *Adverse drug reactions monitoring*. Vol. 2006. Geneva: Author.

Wylie, K. (2008, August 29). Alternative drug sells out. *The Press*.

3 How alcohol marketing engages users with alcohol brand content on Facebook

An Indian and Australian perspective

Himanshu Gupta, Simone Pettigrew, Tina Lam and Robert J. Tait

ABSTRACT

Little work has been conducted to understand how alcohol marketers engage users with their brands' Facebook pages in India and Australia. We aimed to evaluate and compare (i) the types of marketing techniques alcohol marketers utilize to facilitate user engagement on their brands' Facebook pages and (ii) the extent to which users engage with these techniques in two diverse national contexts. We identified the ten most popular alcohol brands on Facebook in India and Australia based on the number of 'likes' for each official brand site. Brand websites and data analytic sources were accessed to collect metrics relating to number of likes, frequency of posts made by alcohol marketers on their brand websites and the resulting comments from fans, and messages relating to responsible drinking. The identified brands accrued substantial user engagement (e.g. Budweiser beer attracted 12.8 million likes in Australia and Foster's beer 802,807 likes in India). The strategies employed were a mix of country-specific (e.g. India: inspirational talks and livelihood skills vs. Australia: posts related to the brand's tradition or heritage) and generic approaches (e.g. alcohol sponsorship of sport, music, and fashion, offering consumption suggestions, organizing competitions, giveaways, and use of memes). This cross-national comparison illustrates that alcohol marketing on Facebook is user-focused and flexible, works with specific national contexts, and capitalizes on the cultural meanings users invoke in their interactions with sites. The study results also demonstrate the potential for brands to engage those under the legal drinking age by delivering alcohol content on Facebook.

Introduction

The considerable time people spend on social networking sites (SNS) has resulted in alcohol marketers investing substantially in online advertising (Nicholls, 2012). Thus, one of the global alcohol industry leaders, Diageo, attributed a 20% increase in the sale of its Smirnoff and Baileys products to increased Facebook marketing (Nhean et al., 2012). Young people engage with social media more than other age groups and thus are more vulnerable to alcohol-related advertising and the harms associated with it (Dobson, 2012). When exposed to alcohol advertisements on SNS, young people can develop pro-drinking attitudes (Alhabash, McAlister, Quilliam, Richards, & Lou, 2015). This is likely to encourage regular alcohol consumption (Jones, Robinson, Barrie, Francis, & Lee, 2016), promote cultures of heavy and risky drinking (Barnes et al., 2016), and increase the risk of developing alcohol-related problems later in life (Hoffman, Pinkleton, Weintraub Austin, & Reyes-Velázquez, 2014).

Supplemental data for this article can be accessed here. [http://dx.doi.org/10.1080/09581596.2017.1318203]

Facebook provides an opportunity for companies to utilize marketing strategies as diverse as their consumer base. Customer segment dissimilarities provide companies with the opportunity to employ different marketing strategies to engage users on Facebook. Cross-national comparisons of Facebook alcohol sites have the potential to illustrate how alcohol marketers use SNS to adapt their online promotional activities to specific cultural contexts. As such, a comparative approach was adopted for this study.

India and Australia have diverse socio-cultural contexts and histories, and are examples of 'dry' and 'wet' drinking cultures. For example, the estimated annual per capita consumption of pure alcohol is 4.3 liters in India compared to 12.2 liters in Australia (World Health Organization [WHO], 2014). There are also country-specific differences in consumption across genders and in preferences for particular beverage categories. In both countries, men drink more than women, although the proportions differ substantially. Annual per capita consumption is estimated at 8 liters for Indian men and 0.5 liters for Indian women, compared to 17 and 7 liters among Australian men and women, respectively (WHO, 2014). Using data on taxed beverages, spirits appear to be the most popular choice in India, whereas beer is most popular in Australia (WHO, 2014).

The discrepancies between the countries can be further observed in the rates of youth drinking. In India, 12% (11% male vs. 1% female) of those aged 15–19 years and 30% (28% male vs. 2% female) of those aged 20–24 years report consuming alcohol (Parasuraman, Kishor, Singh, & Vaidehi, 2009). In comparison, 29% of those aged 12–17 years and 84% of those aged 18–24 years consume alcohol in Australia, with consumption rates being similar for males and females (Australian Institute of Health & Welfare [AIHW], 2014). India has a less developed heavy drinking culture. For example, about 4% of 18–24 year old Indians are classed as 'heavy drinkers', which is defined as consuming at least 40 g of pure alcohol in a single session at least once a month (International Institute for Population Sciences [IIPS], 2003). In contrast, in the same age group, 25% of Australians consume at least 50 g of alcohol in a single sitting, and 15% consume more than 110 g at least once a month (AIHW, 2014).

Further, patterns of alcohol initiation are moving in opposite directions: in Australia, the average age of initiation increased from 14 years in 1998 to 16 years in 2013 (AIHW, 2014), but decreased in India from 19 to 13 years over the past two decades (Prasad, 2009). This trend is concerning for India, as a lowering age of initiation means that more people are at risk of adverse alcohol-related outcomes (Babor et al., 2010).

Alcohol consumption patterns vary with wealth, education, and geographical distribution. In India, alcohol is consumed by about 27% of men and 0.5% of women in the highest wealth quintile and 41% of men and 6% of women in the lowest quintile (IIPS, 2007). While urban and rural Indian men consume alcohol almost equally (31 vs. 33%), a much greater difference is apparent among women by location (0.6% urban vs. 3% rural). Consistent with the wealth quintile findings, populations with low levels of education consume more alcohol than those with high levels of education – 43% men and 4% women with no education compared with 25% men and 0.6% women with the highest level of education (IIPS, 2007). Conversely, those in the top quintile are the most prevalent drinkers in Australia (83% in the top quintile vs. 69% in the lowest quintile; AIHW, 2014). Further, lifetime risky drinking in Australia is more prevalent in remote/very remote (34.9%) than urban (16.7%) areas and among those with post-school qualifications (19.7%) than those without these qualifications (16.0%; AIHW, 2014). These national differences in consumption rates may result from an interplay of socio-cultural norms, such as lower social acceptance of alcohol (Murthy, 2015), religious proscriptions (e.g. lower prevalence of drinking among the 14% of the population in India who identify as Muslims; Census of India, 2011; Murthy, 2015), and the legal drinking age in India ranging from 18–25 years, with sales banned in certain states (Arora et al., 2013).

Facebook is used extensively by Indians and Australians. It is estimated that there are 108 million Facebook users in India (Stastista, 2016), of whom about 50 million are aged 18–24 years and about 12 million are 17 years of age or younger (Nayak, 2014). In 2015, there were an estimated 11 million Australian Facebook users, of whom about 4 million were aged 13–24 years (Stastista, 2016). Given the increasing use of Facebook by alcohol marketers (Nhean et al., 2012), young people who are active on Facebook are at risk of exposure to this marketing. However, work in understanding engagement with alcohol-related content on Facebook is in its infancy. There is a small but growing body of research exploring how Australians engage with such marketing practices and the potential impacts on alcohol consumption behaviors. These include descriptive (Jones & Magee, 2011; Jones et al., 2016) and exploratory studies (Carah, 2014; Carah, Meurk, Males, & Brown, 2017; Dobson, 2012; Lim, Hare, Carrott, & Dietze, 2016). The present study appears to be the first investigating social media marketing of alcohol brands from an Indian perspective. Against this background, this study aims to investigate the extent of user engagement with alcohol brand content and to examine and compare the types of marketing techniques marketers utilize to facilitate user engagement on popular Indian and Australian alcohol brands' Facebook pages.

Methods

Data sourcing

The search strategy (Table 1) was informed by an Australian study of alcohol brands' Facebook pages (Carah, 2014). We compiled a comprehensive list of alcohol brands from key reports on alcohol marketing and the alcohol policy environment in India (Arora et al., 2013; Alcohol brands in India, 2013) and Australia (Lin, 2015; McCusker Centre for Action on Alcohol & Youth, 2014). This list comprised 256 and 287 brands distributed in India and Australia, respectively. In each case we searched for a brand Facebook page. While Facebook is a single, worldwide SNS, alcohol brand Facebook pages are country specific, but users can access these from around the world. Where more than one brand-specific Facebook page was available for a brand, we used the 'switch region tab' to see the India/Australia-specific posts (Winpenny, Marteau, & Nolte, 2014). We also sought a statement such as 'this is the official page' on the 'about' tab on the brand's Facebook page. The absence of this statement excluded the brand from the analysis.

Brands with a local Facebook presence were searched for the number of likes they had received. The ten brands in each country with the highest number were selected. There was no overlap between the brands identified for the two countries, but Diageo owns multiple Indian and Australian brands included in the study (Table 2).

To explore the extent of user engagement, the following information was collected for two months (December 2015–January 2016): the number of posts published and the number of likes, fans, and shares that posts received. Becoming a fan means that one receives content (such as status updates, pictures, etc.) from the brand; liking the page does not generate such content. However, Facebook has recently changed this process so that to become a 'fan' of a page, one simply clicks 'like' on the brand page. Hence, there are 'brand likes' vs. 'post likes' (with the latter referring to liking an individual communication the brand has posted, whether or not one is currently a fan or had liked the entire brand page). For clarity, we have used the legacy term 'fans', in addition to likes. While the number of likes and the year the brand appeared on Facebook were gathered from Facebook-generated metrics, the numbers of fans, posts, and shares were sourced from the Socialbakers website (which provides

Table 1. Search strategy to select the 10 most 'liked' brands in both India and Australia on Facebook.

	India	Australia
Alcohol reports used	• Report on alcohol marketing and regulatory policy environment in India (2013) • Liquor Brands in India (2013)	• MCAAY (2014) • IBIS World Industry Report Beer Manufacturing in Australia (2015) • IBIS World Industry Report Spirit Manufacturing in Australia (2015)
No. of alcohol brands distributed in the country	256	287
Brands with Facebook presence	28	134
Brands with dedicated official Facebook pages	25	67

Table 2. User engagement with Facebook (December 2015–January 2016).

Country	Brand	Beverage category	First year on Facebook	Likes	Fans	Posts (brand-generated)	Shares (user made)
India	Foster's	Beer	2010	802,807	803,339	325	13,949
	Haywards 5000	Beer	2013	699,492	697,415	314	13,245
	Royal Challenge[a]	Whisky	2010	389,049	386,398	256	20,871
	Kingfisher	Beer	2013	376,233	7,288,069	278	23,262
	McDowell's No. 1[a]	Whisky	2012	367,865	378, 915	178	18,466
	Black Dog	Whisky	2010	188,312	189,981	92	1,210
	White Mischief	Vodka	2009	143,119	71,782	71	486
	Breezer	RTD	2011	126,556	629,184	143	12,287
	Vat 69[a]	Whisky	2012	99,075	100,750	87	402
	Blenders Pride	Whisky	2011	9,073	256,066	101	1,768
	Subtotal	–		3,209,754	10,801,899	1,845	85,075
Australia	Budweiser	Beer	2010	12,827,216	42,476	327	23,205
	Smirnoff[a]	Vodka	2009	11,550,463	255,343	234	28,169
	Johnnie Walker[a]	Whisky	2008	11,474,737	136,699	267	36,342
	Corona Extra	Beer	2010	8,815,797	55,424	144	14,231
	Stella Artois	Beer	2012	7,628,921	25,475	123	9,286
	Absolut	Vodka	2009	5,830,061	80,783	132	11,681
	Baileys	Whisky	2009	4,106,013	188,266	111	19,210
	Jägermeister	Liqueur	2010	3,999,889	137,572	145	3,172
	Patron Tequila	Tequila	2009	3,723,251	23,017	102	1,204
	SKYY Vodka	Vodka	2013	3,213,251	26,927	112	2,168
	Subtotal	–	–	73,169,929	297,819	1,686	148,668
	Total	–	–	76,379,683	11,099,718	3,531	233,743

Notes: RTD = ready-to-drink product.
[a]Owned by Diageo.

statistics and metrics for social media websites: Socialbakers, 2016), as these data were not available on the brands' Facebook pages.

Coding process and analysis

Brand-generated posts and user comments were downloaded and analyzed using NVivo10 to facilitate detailed thematic analysis. As the coding process was emergent in nature (i.e. an inductive approach was adopted rather than a deductive approach; Huberman & Miles, 1994), a single coder (the lead author) undertook the coding process. As per Strauss and Corbin (1990), the coding process involved commencing with a priori codes identified from the relevant alcohol literature that were progressively supplemented with codes emerging from the data. The resulting NVivo nodes were interrogated to generate themes, which were subsequently discussed among the members of the research team to refine the final categories.

Additionally, frequency of comments on brands' pages, links to the official brands' websites, links to Twitter/YouTube/Instagram, and messages related to responsible drinking were collected (Winpenny et al., 2014). Numerical data were managed using MS Excel. Ethics approval to access these data was obtained from the Curtin University (ethics approval number: RDHS-239-15).

Results

User engagement

Of the top ten Indian brands, five were whisky, three were beer, one was a ready-to-drink (RTD) rum-based product, and one was a vodka brand. In contrast, three of the top Australian brands were beer, three were vodka, two were whisky, one was tequila, and one was a liqueur. In both India and Australia, the most popular brand was a beer, with 800,000 (Foster's) and 12.8 million (Budweiser) likes, respectively.

Table 2 shows the extensive content brands posted, which was associated with substantial user engagement in the form of likes, fans, posts generated by the brands, and posts shared by the users. The Australian brands accumulated many more likes, had more fans, and more post shares than their Indian equivalents. In some cases, brands with fewer fans had more content sharing. Thus, McDowell's No. 1 had fewer fans and more shares than Foster's, which had more fans and fewer shares. Also, the number of posts generated did not directly correspond to the number of fans and vice-versa. For example, 803,339 fans generated 325 posts for Foster's, whereas Budweiser had 42,476 fans who produced 327 posts.

Content of alcohol marketing

Various techniques were used on the brands' websites to encourage engagement with users. The strategies employed were a mix of country-specific (e.g. India: camaraderie, inspirational talks, and livelihood skills vs. Australia: posts related to the brand's tradition or heritage) and generic approaches (e.g. alcohol sponsorship of sport, music, and fashion, time-and-event-specific drinking, offering consumption suggestions, organizing competitions, giveaways, sexually suggestive content, and use of memes; Tables S1 & S2).

Some of the Australian brands involved creating stories related to users' traditions, cultural heritage, interests, and values. For example, Jägermeister uploaded photos and videos prompting users to celebrate Australia Day by drinking alcohol, and Johnnie Walker and Stella Artois uploaded images of the brands' founding fathers narrating stories about the history of their distilleries/breweries in a specific region. On the other hand, Haywards 5000, a popular Indian brand, promoted several entrepreneurship programs under the name of 'Hauslabuland Academy', where those who had previously benefitted from such programs narrated their own stories, mentioning the brand's name.

Several Indian brands utilized inspirational talks to facilitate interaction with users. Statements such as 'Progress comes when you step outside your comfort zone' (Haywards 5000) and 'Every little thing contributes to great success. #Pause and let's raise a toast to all your victories' (Black Dog) indirectly relate success and hard work to alcohol consumption. Other common themes for Indian brands were camaraderie, togetherness, and acceptance within the users' social networks:

> This leap day, take a giant leap towards friendship and catch up with that long lost friend of yours over a #DaaaaamnColdDaaaaamnCo#Stayrefreshed (Foster's)

> Which is your all-time #No1Yaari gaana? (asking users to post their all-time favourite friendship song) (McDowell's No. 1).

Brands appeared to tap into users' interests and embed those interests into their drinking cultures through such posts. In addition, both Indian and Australian brands utilized Internet memes and modified them to the brand's identity to add humor and 'savviness' to attract users to such content. These posts accrued extensive user engagement in the form of users reproducing multiple meanings of the original posted content. For example, to Jägermeister's meme portraying a majestic stag and a small fox with human bodies with a statement, 'Bigger isn't always better … Introducing … The new 200 milliliters', users readily engaged and responded in several ways including: 'This could be the key to success' and 'Introducing another way to make more money woo'.

Posts also related to promoting brands at cultural, music, fashion, and sporting events. This involved uploading photos/videos taken at events and asking users to narrate their own stories and post pictures relating to celebrating events with drinking. The majority of Australian brands (e.g. Absolut) and several Indian brands (e.g. Black Dog) posted content relating to music festivals or award events sponsored by the brand. References to sports were also popular, with Indian brands capitalizing heavily on cricket and Australian brands associating their products with football, surfing, and tennis. Brands also ran event-related competitions such as singing competitions (e.g. McDowell's No. 1) and prize draws (e.g. Stella Artois). While brands did not directly endorse heavy drinking at events, they provided users with content they could link to their own drinking experiences. In this way, the brands created stories about the events and facilitated the linking of those stories to the users' own drinking cultures.

Some brands promoted their products by placing them in advertisements relating to popular movies. In some cases posts included displaying sexually suggestive content. For instance, White Mischief posted images of attractive women in revealing clothing at various brand-sponsored events.

Brands also posted content depicting brand images/logos on products such as caps and other clothing. Budweiser asked Australian Facebook users to check into events sponsored by the brand and to enter a prize draw to receive a free cap with a Budweiser logo. Users reacted enthusiastically to these posts: 'Yes please, where can I get my hands on one of these?' and posting their pictures with those caps on, saying 'UH OOOOH!!! Thanks Budweiser [for the cap]'. Similarly, the Breezer Facebook page featured posts offering free music CDs bearing its logo.

Both Indian and Australian brands posted images/videos suggesting specific methods of consuming their products. These included demonstrations of cocktail and/or food recipes. Examples include 'Match this loco tropical weather with a delicious Coco Loco!' (Smirnoff) and 'Baileys Cheesecake with Caramel Sauce – mesmerising isn't it?' (Baileys). Users readily engaged with these posts and subsequently shared their own recipes on brands' walls. Thus, the brands provided users with information that encouraged further communication and interaction by users. This strategy appeared to target users' interests and to embed the consumption of the products within those interests.

Brands published posts suggesting drinking at a particular time or event, such as after work, on weekends and public holidays, at festivals, and during brand-sponsored tours:

> Saturdays are for Sunshine, Smirnoff, Shorts and Sandals. #SLIPSLOPSLAP' (Smirnoff)

> Experience the Good Times all around, with #KF360Cities! This time we take you on a tour of Pondicherry, with its golden sands and French colonial architecture, in 360°! #360Video (Kingfisher)

> Where will you be raising your chalice this Australia Day? (Stella Artois)

User responses to the Black Dog post about taking a pause from work by consuming whisky included comments such as 'I should be doing this right now. Apparently there's some rule about not being under the influence of alcohol while working. I do my best work when I'm drinking'. Such content appeared to be aligned with users' interests, hence increasing the affinity between brands and users and prompting them to drink.

Some of the brands also published posts relating to sexually suggestive content in the context of time- and event-specific drinking: Budweiser uploaded photos of women wearing swimsuits, lying by a pool, and enjoying a glass of beer. These types of images generated numerous comments from users such as 'Find the hot chicks then get some beer'.

Nine of the Australian brands had a link to DrinkWise (an alcohol industry funded organization) on their Facebook pages. In contrast, five of the Indian brands provided information about responsible consumption, such as messages related to drinking and driving. However, none of the brands appeared to have links to non-industry affiliated responsible drinking information sources such as government websites.

Discussion

Although India has a much larger population (Census of India, 2011) and many more Facebook users than Australia (Stastista, 2016), interaction in terms of likes on alcohol brand Facebook pages was higher for Australia. The reason for the lesser user engagement for the Indian brands is unclear, but could be an interplay of various socio-cultural norms, such as lower social acceptance of alcohol (Murthy, 2015), religious proscriptions (Murthy, 2015), significant gender differences in alcohol consumption (World Health Organization, 2014), and a less-developed drinking culture (Rathod, Nadkarni, Bhana, & Shidhaye, 2015). There are fewer cultural inhibitions to prevent users from engaging with brands in the Australian context, which is likely to largely account for the greater user engagement observed for the Australian brand pages. It is argued that the greater the number of fans a brand has, the greater the chances that the brand's page will be seen by the Facebook friends of that fan, hence further increasing user engagement with the brand (Carah, 2014). Thus, becoming a 'fan' is likely to be more powerful than 'liking' in the minds of one's Facebook friends.

We identified country-specific techniques employed to engage users. These included some of the Indian brands explicitly utilizing and embedding camaraderie and togetherness into the users' drinking cultures. This is possibly attributed to users' leisure-driven engagement with Facebook that feeds into the 'aspirational' quality of Facebook to reach out to the disenfranchised in India (Kumar, 2014), and thus increasing the brands' reach to this part of the community (especially younger men) that accesses Facebook typically on mobile phones (Kumar, 2014). Some of the Australian brands associated their products with users' cultures and interests. Associating 'belongingness' to a common heritage, as was done by the Australian brands, could potentially be the Australian version of the Indian 'togetherness'. Such practices appeared to be attempts to localize the brands and make them part of real communities, regions, and livelihoods.

Associations between higher alcohol consumption and lower education and socioeconomic status in India (IIPS, 2007) could potentially explain the instances of 'inspirational' marketing content and the specific emphasis on offering 'livelihood skills' identified on the Indian brands' sites. These country-specific examples could reflect underlying differences in the users attracted to the brands, differences in the brands' ability to generate content that fans wanted to share, or differences between 'individualistic' and 'collectivistic' cultures in the propensity to share and engage with SNS content (Jackson & Wang, 2013).

Demographic information was not available on brands' pages and thus we were unable to determine the ages and genders of those engaging with the brands. However, the identified engagement strategies utilized by both the Indian and Australian brands (i.e. competitions, prize draws, free tickets to music events) suggest young people were being targeted given evidence linking the popularity of such strategies with young people (Weaver, Wright, Dietze, & Lim, 2016). Such strategies also do not always conform to the existing Alcohol Beverages Advertising Code (ABAC) in Australia (Weaver et al., 2016), hence necessitate effective implementation of these guidelines, particularly in relation to younger Facebook users. Further, the Advertising Standard Council of India (ASCI) does not restrict

Internet-based alcohol advertising (Advertising Standards Council of India [ASCI], 2013), hence alcohol advertising via social media is largely unregulated and rampant in India, as evident from this study.

We found that brands accumulated extensive likes on their Facebook pages. For example, Budweiser beer accrued 12.8 million likes within Australia, a country with a total population of around 24 million (Australian Bureau of Statistics, 2016). Some alcohol brands create multiple artificial identities and fake profiles on Facebook to facilitate the widespread dissemination of their messages (Dobson, 2012). Thus, although the brands in this study accrued a substantial number of likes, this technique makes the 'real' popularity of their Facebook presence uncertain. Also, we could not determine if users were followers of just one particular brand or whether they follow multiple brands, so the total number of people exposed to the alcohol-related content is unknown.

The lack of effective age restrictions on social media access (and thus potential exposure to marketing) combined with emerging evidence that links exposure to alcohol advertising with earlier or greater alcohol use by young people has urgent policy implications (Gupta, Pettigrew, Lam, & Tait, 2016). SNS marketing should be required to abide by the same requirements as television advertising because the potential effects on young people are comparable (Dobson, 2012). This is likely to be difficult because where posts are not of interest to users, they can be quickly removed from a brand's newsfeed (Carah, 2014). This flexibility means that brands can rapidly modify content in response to users' engagement (or non-engagement) in a way that cannot be done in traditional advertisements. The marketing strategies described in this paper may also be used over other networking platforms (e.g. Instagram and Twitter). As such, future research may seek to compare strategies used to target the same audience over multiple platforms. Finally, there was no brand overlap between countries in our sample, so it may be useful to examine how individual brands are marketed across different countries.

Some limitations should be considered when interpreting results of this study. The most important is the inclusion of only two countries in a cross-country comparison and the limited time period for data collection that could have different seasonal characteristics for each country. In addition, some selection bias could result from identifying the brands with the highest number of Facebook likes rather than using a random selection from all eligible brands. Given the gender disparities in alcohol use in India (IIPS, 2007), an analysis by gender would also be of interest, but it was not possible to identify this in the current data-set.

A further consideration is that this study undertook a largely exploratory approach to report the techniques that alcohol brands employ to engage consumers on Facebook. However, as alcohol marketing on social media represents a new challenge and work on this topic is in its infancy, an exploratory approach was required to inform future analyses that can aim to produce more generalizable results. In particular, additional cross-national comparisons of this kind are warranted to demonstrate how alcohol marketers use SNS to adapt their online promotional activities to specific cultural contexts.

Disclosure statement

No potential conflict of interest was reported by the authors.

Funding

The National Drug Research Institute at Curtin University is supported by funding from the Australian Government under the Substance Misuse Prevention and Service Improvement Grants Fund. This work was supported by the Curtin Faculty of Health Science International Research Scholarship (HG); a fellowship from the Western Australian Health Promotion Foundation (Healthway; TL), and a Curtin University Research Fellowship (RJT).

ORCID

Himanshu Gupta (iD) http://orcid.org/0000-0003-1952-3816

References

Advertising Standards Council of India. (2013). *The code for self-regulation in advertising*. Retrieved from http://www. ascionline.org/images/pdf/asci_code1new.pdf

Alhabash, S., McAlister, A. R., Quilliam, E. T., Richards, J. I., & Lou, C. (2015). Alcohol's getting a bit more social: When alcohol marketing messages on Facebook increase young adults' intentions to imbibe. *Mass Communication and Society, 18*, 350–375. doi:10.1080/15205436.2014.945651

Arora, M., Dahiya, P., Nazar, G., Gupta, H., Singh, D., Sahoo, P., … Chatterjee, M. (2013). Alcohol marketing and regulatory policy environment in India. A Report. Public Health Foundation of India. New Delhi, India: PHFI. Retrieved from http:// iogt.org/wp-content/uploads/2013/12/PHFI-Alcohol-Industry-Report.pdf

Australian Bureau of Statistics. (2016). *Census Data*. Retrieved from http://www.abs.gov.au/ausstats/abs@. nsf/0/1647509ef7e25faaca2568a900154b63?OpenDocument

Australian Institute of Health and Welfare. (2014). *National drug strategy household survey detailed report 2013* (Drug statistics series no. 28. Cat. no. PHE 183). Canberra, Australia: Author.

Babor, T. F., Caetano, R., Casswell, S., Edwards, G., Giesbrecht, N., Graham, K., … Rossow, I. (2010). Alcohol: No ordinary commodity – a summary of the 2nd ed. *Addiction, 105*, 769–779. doi:10.1111/j.1360-0443.2010.02945.x

Barnes, H. M., McCreanor T., Goodwin, I., Lyons, A., Griffin, C., & Hutton, F. (2016). Alcohol and social media: Drinking and drunkenness while online. *Critical Public Health, 26*, 62–76. doi:10.1080/09581596.2015.1058921

Carah, N. (2014). *Like, comment, share alcohol brand activity on Facebook*. Deakin: Foundation for Alcohol Research and Education, University of Queensland. Retrieved from http://fare.org.au/wp-content/uploads/research/Facebook-and-alcohol-advertising-report.pdf

Carah, N., Meurk, C., Males, M., & Brown, J. (2017). Emerging social media 'platform' approaches to alcohol marketing: A comparative analysis of the activity of the top 20 Australian alcohol brands on Facebook (2012–2014). *Critical Public Health, 1*–11. doi:10.1080/09581596.2017.1282154

Dobson, C. (2012). *Alcohol marketing and young people: Time for a new policy agenda*. Kingston: AMA. Retrieved from https:// ama.com.au/sites/default/files/documents/alcohol_marketing_young_people.pdf

Gupta, H., Pettigrew, S., Lam, T., & Tait, R. J. (2016). A systematic review of the impact of exposure to Internet-based alcohol-related content on young people's alcohol use behaviours. *Alcohol and Alcoholism, 51*, 763–771. doi:10.1093/alcalc/ agw050

Hoffman, E. W., Pinkleton, B. E., Weintraub Austin, E., & Reyes-Velázquez, W. (2014). Exploring college students' use of general and alcohol-related social media and their associations with alcohol-related behaviors. *Journal of American College Health, 62*, 328–335. doi:10.1080/07448481.2014.902837

Huberman, A. M., & Miles, M. B. (1994). Data management and analysis methods. In N. K. Denzin & Y. S. Lincoln (Eds.), *Handbook of qualitative research* (pp. 428–444). Thousand Oaks, CA: Sage.

International Institute for Population Sciences and Macro International. (2007). *National Family Health Survey (NFHS-3) 2005–06*. New Delhi: Ministry of Health and Family Welfare, Government of India. Retrieved from http://www.measuredhs. com/pubs/pdf/SR128/SR128.pdf

International Institute for Population Sciences, World Health Organization. (2003). Health system performance assessment. World Health Survey, 2003, India. Geneva: India-WR Office. Retrieved from http://www.who.int/healthinfo/survey/ whs_hspa_book.pdf

Jackson, L. A., & Wang, J. L. (2013). Cultural differences in social networking site use: A comparative study of China and the United States. *Computers in Human Behavior, 29*, 910–921. doi:10.1016/j.chb.2012.11.024

Jones, S., & Magee, C. (2011). Exposure to alcohol advertising and alcohol consumption among Australian adolescents. *Alcohol and Alcoholism, 46*, 630–637. doi:10.1093/alcalc/agr080

Jones, S. C., Robinson, L., Barrie, L., Francis, K., & Lee, J. K. (2016). Association between young Australian's drinking behaviours and their interactions with alcohol brands on Facebook: Results of an Online Survey. *Alcohol and Alcoholism, 1*–17. doi:10.1093/alcalc/agv113

Kumar, N. (2014). Facebook for self-empowerment? A study of Facebook adoption in urban India. *New Media and Society, 16*, 1122–1137. doi:10.1177/1461444814543999

Lim, M. S. C., Hare, J. D., Carrott, E. R., & Dietze, P. M. (2016). An investigation of strategies used in alcohol brand marketing and alcohol-related health promotion on Facebook. *Digital Health, 2*, 1–7. doi:10.1177/2055207616647305

Lin, R. (2015). Lifted spirits: Successful boutique distilleries entice new industry entrants. IBIS World Industry Report C1213 Beer/Spirit Manufacturing in Australia. Retrieved from http://clients1.ibisworld.com.au/reports/au/industry/default. aspx?entid=116; http://clients1.ibisworld.com.au/reports/au/industry/default.aspx?entid=118

List of alcohol brands in India and their distillery name. (2013). Retrieved from http://www.theboozeguru.com/liquorbrands. htm

McCusker Centre for Action on Alcohol and Youth. (2014). A Guide to the Alcohol Industry. Retrieved from https://mcaay. org.au/assets/publications/industry-guides/mcaay_aguidetothealcoholindustry_feb2014-final.pdf

Murthy, P. (2015). Culture and alcohol use in India. *World Association of Cultural Psychiatry*, 27–39.

Nayak, V. (2014). 92 million Facebook users make India the second largest country. Retrieved from http://dazeinfo. com/2014/01/07/facebook-inc-fb-india-demographic-users-2014/

Nhean, S., Nyborn, J., Hinchey, D., Valerio, H., Kinzel, K., … Jernigan, D. H. (2012). The frequency of company sponsored alcohol brand-related sites on Facebook. *Substance Use Misuse, 49*, 779–782. doi: 10.3109/10826084.2014.880177

Nicholls, J. (2012). Everyday, everywhere: Alcohol marketing and social media – current trends. *Alcohol and Alcoholism, 47*, 486–493. doi:10.1093/alcalc/ags043

Office of the Registrar General & Census Commissioner, Ministry of Home Affairs, Government of India. (2011). Census of India. Retrieved from http://www.censusindia.gov.in/2011census/C-01.html

Parasuraman, S., Kishor, S., Singh, S. K., & Vaidehi, Y. (2009). *National Family Health Survey (NFHS-3), India, 2005–06*. Mumbai: International Institute for Population Sciences. Retrieved from http://www.rchiips.org/NFHS/youth_report_for_website_18sep09.pdf

Prasad, R. (2009). Alcohol use on the rise in India. *The Lancet, 373*, 17–18. PubMed PMID: 19125444. Epub 2009/01/07. eng.

Rathod, S. D., Nadkarni, A., Bhana, A., & Shidhaye, R. (2015). Epidemiological features of alcohol use in rural India: A population-based cross-sectional study. *British Medical Journal Open, 5*, e009802. doi:10.1136/bmjopen-2015-009802

Socialbakers. (2016). Retrieved from http://www.socialbakers.com/statistics/facebook/pages/total/australia/brands/alcohol/; http://www.socialbakers.com/statistics/facebook/pages/total/india/brands/alcohol/

Stastista. (2016). Retrieved from http://www.statista.com/statistics/304827/number-of-facebook-users-in-india/; http://www.statista.com/statistics/304862/number-of-facebook-users-in-australia/

Strauss, A., & Corbin, J. (1990). *Basics of qualitative research*. Thousand Oaks, CA: Sage.

Weaver, E. R. N., Wright, C. J. C., Dietze, P. M., & Lim, M. S. C. (2016). 'A drink that makes you feel happier, relaxed and loving': Young people's perceptions of alcohol advertising on Facebook. *Alcohol and Alcoholism, 51*, 481–486. doi:10.1093/alcalc/agv134

Winpenny, E. M., Marteau, T. M., & Nolte, E. (2014). Exposure of children and adolescents to alcohol marketing on social media websites. *Alcohol and Alcoholism, 49*, 154–159. doi:10.1093/alcalc/agt174

World Health Organization. (2014). *Global status report on alcohol and health*. Geneva, Switzerland: WHO. Retrieved from http://apps.who.int/iris/bitstream/10665/112736/1/9789240692763_eng.pdf

Table S1 Alcohol marketing content on the 10 most popular alcohol brands with an Indian Facebook presence

	Indian Brands (in order of popularity by likes)				
	Foster's	Haywards 5000	Royal Challenge	Kingfisher	McDowell's No. 1
'Like' button	x	x	x	x	x
Video advert	x	-	x	x	x
Competitions/ giveaways	x	-	x	x	x
Alcohol sale links	-	-	-	-	-
Examples of content on brand's Facebook page	• Travel • On tour party videos • Comedy • TESD • Memes • Camaraderie	• Entrepreneur-ship skills • TESD • Camaraderie • Wisdom talks	• Sports • Travel • Cocktail recipes • TESD • Sexual content • Festival celebration • Memes	• Sports • Music festivals • Travel • On tour party videos • Festival celebration • Memes • Consumption suggestions • Fashion • TESD • Sexual content	• Sports • Camaraderie • Prize draw • Memes • Singing competitions
Frequency of brand comments on wall	> weekly	> weekly	> weekly	> weekly	> weekly
Responsible drinking messages	x	-	x	-	-
Link to official website	-	x	x	x	x
Link to Twitter	x	-	-	-	x
Link to YouTube	-	-	-	-	x
Link to Instagram	-	-	-	-	x

	Indian Brands continued (in order of popularity by likes)				
	Black Dog	White Mischief	Breezer	VAT 69	Blenders Pride
'Like' button	x	x	x	x	x
Video advert	x	-	-	-	-
Competitions/ giveaways	x	x	x	-	-
Alcohol sale links	-	-	-	-	-
Examples of content on brand's Facebook page	• Music festivals • Comedy • Luxury • Food recipes • Camaraderie/ Togetherness • Inspirational talks • TESD	• Cocktail recipes • Music festivals • Comedy • Sports • Travel • TESD • Memes • Sexual content	• Music festivals • TESD • Food recipes • Memes • Comedy • Travel	• Cocktail/food recipes • Memes • Camaraderie • Memes • Inspirational talks • Famous quotes from Bollywood movies	• Cocktail recipes • Meme • Festival celebration • Memes • Fashion
Frequency of brand comments on wall	> weekly	> weekly	> weekly	Weekly	> weekly

	Indian Brands continued (in order of popularity by likes)				
	Black Dog	White Mischief	Breezer	VAT 69	Blenders Pride
Responsible drinking messages	x	x	-	x	-
Link to official website	x	x	x	-	x
Link to Twitter	-	x	x	-	-
Link to YouTube	-	x	x	-	-
Link to Instagram	-	-	-	-	-

TESD=Time- and Event-Specific drinking
X=content present; -=content absent
>weekly=more than weekly

Table S2 Alcohol marketing content on the 10 most popular alcohol brands having Australian Facebook presence

	Australian Brands (in order of popularity by likes)				
	Budweiser	Smirnoff	Johnnie Walker	Corona Extra	Stella Artois
'Like' button	x	x	x	x	x
Video advert	x	x	x	x	x
Competitions/ giveaways	x	x	x	x	x
Alcohol sale links	-	-	-	-	-
Examples of content on brand's Facebook page	• Sports • Music festivals • Travel • On tour party videos • Comedy • Posts related to the brand's tradition or heritage • Contests • Sexual content	• Music festivals • Travel • On tour party videos • Cocktail recipes • Contests • Festival celebration • TESD	• Music festivals • Travel • Cocktail recipes • On tour party videos • TESD • Fashion • Motivational videos (e.g. 'Keep walking', 'Be joyous') • Advertisements related to movies • Posts related to the brand's tradition or heritage	• Sports • Music festivals • Travel	• Sports • Advertisements related to movies • Prize draw • Festival celebration • Posts related to the brand's tradition or heritage
Frequency of brand comments on wall	Weekly	> weekly	> weekly	> weekly	Daily
Link to official website	-	x	x	x	x
Link to DrinkWise website	x	x	x	x	x
Link to Twitter	-	-	-	-	-
Link to YouTube	-	-	-	-	-
Link to Instagram	-	x	x	x	-

	Australian Brands continued (in order of popularity by likes)				
	Absolut	**Baileys**	**Jägermeister**	**Patron Tequila**	**SKYY Vodka**
'Like' button	x	x	x	x	x
Video advert	x	-	x	x	-
Competitions/ giveaways	x	x	x	x	-
Alcohol sale links	-	-	-	-	-
Examples of content on brand's Facebook page	• Cocktail recipes • Music festivals • Advertisements related to movies • On tour party videos	• Cocktail recipes • Fashion festivals	• Music festivals/ awards • Cultural (e.g. Australia Day) • TESD • Sports • Meme • Festival celebration • Travel	• Cocktail recipes • Posts related to the brand's tradition or heritage • Music festivals/ awards • Meme • Sexual content	• Music festivals • Cocktail recipes • Meme • Festival celebration • Travel • Sexual content

	Australian Brands (in order of popularity by likes)				
Frequency of brand comments on wall	Weekly	> weekly	> weekly	> weekly	> weekly
Link to official website	-	x	x	x	x
Link to DrinkWise website	x	x	x	x	-
Link to Twitter	-	-	-	-	-
Link to YouTube	-	-	-	-	-
Link to Instagram	-	x	x	x	x

DrinkWise=an alcohol industry funded organization on responsible drinking

4 'To drink or not to drink'

Media framing of evidence and debate about alcohol consumption in pregnancy

Kerry McCallum and Kate Holland

ABSTRACT

The issue of women's consumption of alcohol during pregnancy has gained increasing public attention in Australia in recent years. This article examines the framing of the issue in news media and pregnancy and parenting websites during 2013–2014, with particular attention to the two most prominent frames of 'contested evidence and advice' and 'women's rights'. Public health guidelines in Australia, as elsewhere, advise women that not drinking during pregnancy is the safest option, but debate continues to surround the evidence to support this advice and its impact. This article considers these guidelines in the context of critical public health scholarship highlighting the intensification of discourses of health, risk, and responsibility in relation to pregnancy and maternal practices. Newly published scientific research provided a key source of news about the risks associated with alcohol consumption during pregnancy, with stories reporting on studies that variously identified evidence of harm, or no harm, to the fetus. In the context of the 'women's rights' frame, consuming alcohol during pregnancy was not constructed primarily as a matter of scientific research or expert opinion but as one of many social practices women negotiate during pregnancy. It foregrounded the rights of women to make their own decisions about alcohol consumption. The deployment of these two frames in mediated public discussion of the issue reflects the inconclusiveness of evidence about the risks of low to moderate consumption and shows women critically engaging with public health advice in the context of the numerous directives they are inundated with during pregnancy.

Introduction

The issue of women's consumption of alcohol during pregnancy has gained increasing public attention in Australia in recent years. For example, in 2015 Australia's premier current affairs journalism programme, *Four Corners*, investigated the harms of Fetal Alcohol Spectrum Disorder (FASD) (ABC, 2015). The 'Hidden Harm' programme raised the alarm about the prevalence of FASD in the Australian community and presented evidence that FASD can be caused by low amounts of fetal exposure to alcohol.[1] The programme was wide ranging in its exploration of the issue, delving into the social and individual determinants and consequences of the disability, including the vulnerability of children and adults with FASD in the justice system. Significantly, 'Hidden Harm' privileged women's narratives of disclosure about drinking in pregnancy, as well as those of children affected by FASD, and acknowledged Australia's drinking culture. It discussed the experiences of Indigenous and non-Indigenous families and reported that the burden of FASD is predominantly in the white middle class. This particular journalistic genre allowed for a considered and nuanced exploration of a complex and multifaceted health issue. In this article, we examine how alcohol consumption during pregnancy is more typically framed in Australian news and popular media.

In Australia, the National Health and Medical Research Council's *Guidelines to Reduce Health Risks from Drinking Alcohol* (the Guidelines) counsel that for women who are pregnant, planning pregnancy, or breastfeeding, not drinking is the safest option (NHMRC, 2009). The NHMRC is supported in its communication of the abstinence message by the health bureaucracy, the medical community, and public health advocacy organisations such as the Foundation for Alcohol Research and Education (FARE). The health communication logic here is that news media, with their influential 'effects' on individual behaviours, are a powerful tool available to public health agencies to transmit the abstinence message and change individual behaviours (Leask, Hooker, & King, 2010). However, there has been little research critically analysing the relationships between scientific research findings, public health guidelines and media reporting in the construction of public knowledge about the consumption of alcohol during pregnancy. Our recent research found that women draw on an abundance of complex and frequently contested advice during pregnancy, with news media one important source of information along with medical practitioners, social media networks, and families and friends (Holland, McCallum, & Blood, 2015; Holland, McCallum, & Walton, 2016). While the impacts of news media reporting are mediated by a variety of factors, it forms a crucial element of public understanding of health issues.

This article examines how news and popular health media in Australia frame the government's unequivocal advice that women should abstain from alcohol during pregnancy. We first analyse government-sponsored pregnancy guidelines in the context of critical risk theory and the governance of women's bodies (Lupton, 2012). We then consider the concept of 'biomediatization' (Briggs & Hallin, 2016) to theorize the intimacy between public health and journalism in the co-construction of public health discourse. We outline the constructionist news frame analysis research methodology (Van Gorp, 2007) that allowed us to explore the interplay between context, source, and journalist in the production of news texts, and to identify five contested frames used to tell the alcohol and pregnancy story.

Inconsistent guidelines and unequivocal messaging

Despite an apparently unequivocal public health advocacy message, debate continues to surround the advice provided to women about drinking alcohol when pregnant the evidence to support it, and its impact. Increasing scientific knowledge about the hazards of alcohol to the unborn child and the devastating impacts of FASD on a small proportion of the population drives public health campaigns urging women not to drink alcohol in pregnancy (Elliott, 2014). Research shows that some women do not abstain from alcohol while pregnant (Callinan & Room, 2012; Colvin, Payne, Parsons, Kurinczuk, & Bower, 2007; Peadon et al., 2011; Powers et al., 2010), while there is also evidence that, since 2007, the proportion of Australian women consuming alcohol during pregnancy has declined and the proportion of women abstaining has risen (AIHW, 2014).

In the context of these debates, most Western countries have developed official guidelines advising women on desired pregnancy behaviours. Australia's Guidelines were updated in 2009 and represent a precautionary approach based on limitations of the existing evidence and the impossibility of setting a 'safe' or 'no-risk' level (Keane, 2009, 2013; NHMRC, 2009). The document notes that the abstinence message is 'more conservative' than previous recommendations (ibid, p. 7). However, it is broadly consistent with advice given by health authorities in the United States, Canada, New Zealand, Finland, Denmark, Norway, Sweden, and Switzerland. The UK Department of Health guidelines are more equivocal in the advice they provide to women who do choose to drink during pregnancy (see Donnelly, 2015). At the extreme end of the spectrum, the US Centres for Disease Control recently advised that all women should abstain from alcohol during their childbearing years (CDC, 2016).

Critical feminist and risk approaches to public health position contemporary debates about alcohol and pregnancy as a key element of the 'risk society' (Beck, 1992). Lupton (2013, p. 246) argues that under neoliberalism '[b]oth pregnant women and their fetuses have become biomedical subjects, their bodies defined, given meaning and regulated by the discourses of biomedicine'. State-produced texts, such as the NHMRC Guidelines, can be understood as a form of social control reinforcing a discourse of individual responsibility of the mother, who is simultaneously the protector and greatest threat to the potential citizen (see Keane, 2013). Official guidelines and their associated health education and promotion messages tend to ignore the social and cultural factors that intersect with alcohol use and the burden of its harms (Hunting & Browne, 2012). Their 'aura of objectivity' also masks the choices they reflect about which risks to emphasize, and the abstinence advice has been criticized for formalizing a connection between uncertainty and danger (Keane, 2013, p. 156; Lowe & Lee, 2010; Lyerly et al., 2009). It is argued that in concert with health authorities, news media play a key role in intensifying discourses of health, risk, and responsibility in relation to pregnancy and maternal practices such as alcohol consumption (Day, Gough, & McFadden, 2004; Keane, 2013).

Journalism, public health, and the reporting of alcohol and pregnancy

A media studies approach extends the focus from the agencies of public health promotion to the media institutions and professional journalists who work with public health, medical and science 'experts' and lay audiences to represent complex scientific knowledge (Briggs & Hallin, 2016). Public health authorities rely on news and popular media to transmit the abstinence message to pregnant women and their communities in the expectation of behavioural change (Foundation for Alcohol Research and Education [FARE], 2016; Leask et al., 2010). Journalists also rely on new research findings and public health guidelines as 'authoritative' and relatively easily accessible and trusted sources of health news. In this regard, recent research by Briggs and Hallin (2016; see also Holland, 2017) is useful to move beyond the constructed binaries of autonomous domains of science and journalism. They argue that the two cultures are deeply interdependent. While journalism has become increasingly 'biomedicalized', the 'biomediatization' of health and medicine means they are fundamentally shaped by their interactions with the media (2016, p. 12). The phenomenon of mediatization occurs when changes in the media, on the one hand, impact on the operation of other fields (Couldry & Hepp, 2013). As news media organisations face revenue and resourcing pressures, employing fewer journalists to undertake investigative reporting, public health organisations employ more media professionals to actively structure information and produce content for journalistic consumption that fits news formats and logics (McCallum, & Waller, 2017). According to Briggs and Hallin (2016), the result is that health journalists no longer simply report health news but co-produce it with medical, scientific, public health, and government actors. As public health communicators increasingly adopt the logics and routines of news media to get their message across they may gloss over the complexities and contingencies of scientific knowledge. This increases the imperative to closely study the content of news, particularly the frames through which journalists tell complex health stories.

Women's alcohol consumption has attracted increasing media attention in the past decade (Day et al., 2004; Gentile, 2011). Bogren's (2011) study of gender and alcohol in the Swedish press found that reports emphasized a zero tolerance approach to alcohol consumption in pregnancy even as they noted that the evidence was inconclusive. This study also found that the press constructs responsible mothers as those who avoid alcohol completely. Similarly, Day et al.'s (2004) study found that media reports about alcohol risks during pregnancy function to create a dichotomy between women who do not drink as responsible and those who do, even the smallest amount, as irresponsible and 'bad' mothers. These authors argue that media reporting equates femininity with motherhood and that this is 'a central reason why women's drinking has and continues to be subject to scrutiny and moral panic' (Day et al., 2004, p. 178; see also Armstrong, 1998; Bell, McNaughton, & Salmon, 2009; Leppo, 2012; Lupton, 2011, 2013). Rodriguez's (2013) Australian study of print media portrayals of FASD and alcohol consumption during pregnancy identified a generally sympathetic discourse about people with FASD (the FASD victim frame), whereas stories treated women who drank during pregnancy more variably; some were sympathetic, some were neutral, and others were critical. Our study builds on these findings but extends the scope of investigation to take account of the breadth and diversity of the contemporary news environment.

Research approach: news framing in a changing media context

Framing is a useful theoretical and methodological tool for the analysis of media content in public discussion of alcohol consumption during pregnancy. The frame is the 'organizing principle' (Reese, 2007, p. 150) through which an issue is presented in a media text, reflecting journalistic decisions and professional routines (Reese, 2007; see also D'Angelo, 2002). According to De Vreese (2014, p. 137) 'the frame highlights the active role of journalists in constructing news stories, a process which is at the core of mediatization'. Our research is informed by the constructionist approach to framing that emphasizes the representation of an issue within its political and social contexts (Van Gorp, 2007). This is particularly useful for analysing texts in highly mediatized contexts as it can take into account the role of news sources, prominent voices, and audiences in a story.

Sources of news such as governments, health experts and other interest groups engage in framing activities as they seek to strategically advance their particular problem definitions and proposed solutions (Gamson & Modigliani, 1989). This approach sees frames as cultural phenomena that 'carry excess meaning', 'inviting the public to view the world and social relations in a certain way', and this can have implications for public opinion and policy responses (Holmes, 2009, p. 225). For example, focusing on individuals as personally to blame can obscure the role of social and cultural conditions and potentially contribute to stigma and constrained policy responses (Carlisle & Hanlon, 2007; Rail & Beausoleil, 2003). Conversely, framing an issue within its wider social, political, and economic context may encourage individuals to recognize constraints on individual choice and responsibility (Hansen & Gunter, 2007; Shugart, 2011). Finally, audiences also actively engage in issue framing and may share or resist other frames based on their interests, beliefs, experiences, and desires (Van Gorp, 2007).

With the advent of digital and social media platforms has come a parallel decline in the authority of news media and journalism to articulate the public conversation (Watkins et al., 2016). Public health advocates and medical practitioners can communicate directly with their audiences or clients using websites and social and mobile media, reducing the reliance on journalists to translate complex messages. The role of the journalist as gatekeeper is further diluted through the convergence of commercial public relations and journalism for the production of news content (Turner, 2016). News audiences are increasingly fluid and fractured, with less loyalty to media brands, and social media has fundamentally altered the consumption of news resulting in a situation whereby news on popular media sites, shared through social media such as Facebook and Twitter, can generate extensive public discussion outside of institutional news media sites (Watkins et al., 2016). In the context of this changing media environment it could be argued that the framing paradigm, with its focus on 'institutional' media as the locus of the public sphere and its inherent assumptions of mass media dominance and a static audience, has passed its use by date. We argue that the changing media environment challenges but does not undermine the framing paradigm. We contend that it is more important than ever to provide analyses of mediated discussion about an issue. Journalism, taken in its broadest sense, remains a key site of public health discussion, particularly where governments have an interest in funding public health campaigns to shift behaviours (Fogarty & Chapman, 2012).

Methodology: qualitative news framing analysis

The aim of our study was to understand how Australia's media represents drinking alcohol in pregnancy and how they portray official guidelines and scientific debate on the issue. We followed the qualitative framing methodology developed by Blood and Holland (2004) to discern the routine, strategic and contested frames in media stories (Blood, Dare, McCallum, Holland, & Pirkis, 2008). The research team identified news and popular media coverage of alcohol and pregnancy between 1 January 2013 and 31 October 2014 from four newspapers: *The Australian*, *The Sydney Morning Herald*, *The Daily Telegraph* and

Canberra Times, as well as television news and current affairs programmes, and articles from pregnancy and parenting websites, both Australian and international, including *Essential Baby*, *Mother and Baby*, *Bubhub*, *Mommyish* and *motherinc*. News stories were also identified from *Crikey* and ABC's *The Pulse*. We deliberately chose a wide range of media, rather than only 'hard news', to reflect the convergence of media platforms and content in the digital age.

These media items constituted the database from which our figures for story counts are drawn. The Factiva and TVNews databases were used to find news items originating from online, print media, and television news and current affairs, with search engines used for news web pages and pregnancy and parenting sites. Media items were identified using the search terms alcohol* AND pregnancy*. Items were then filtered for relevance to the consumption of alcohol during pregancy and entered into the custom-built 'Alcohol and Pregnancy' database. A total of 110 media items were collected and recorded, and each item was coded across a range of factors, including source, genre, topic, and key spokesperson. Our sample comprised: 60 newspaper stories (print and online), 36 articles from parenting and pregnancy websites, and 14 television news or current affairs stories. While this data-set does not represent a generalisable sample of all news media coverage of the issue, it provides a comprehensive snapshot of dimensions of media interest and is indicative of public discussion around this health topic. Following the preliminary mapping and coding exercise, we conducted a close reading of each media item in concert with existing academic literature. Acknowledging the co-production of pregnancy news between actors in the public health domain we paid particular attention to the sponsors of different frames, dominant voices, overall tone, and key message indicated in the headline.

Framing alcohol in pregnancy

Our initial coding found that 59% of stories mentioned FASD, 40% mentioned that women were advised to abstain from drinking alcohol while pregnant, and 18% mentioned the NHMRC Guidelines. On the other hand, 26% of stories stated or implied that a certain amount of alcohol in pregnancy was not harmful; even if that same article went on to quote the NHMRC's abstinence advice. This initial coding provided valuable baseline information for our qualitative framing analysis. We identified five key frames across the corpus of media texts: 'contested evidence and advice'; 'women's rights'; 'FASD crisis'; 'blame risk-taking mothers'; and 'community responsibility'. Our framing analysis found that apart from a sub-set of stories about FASD in Indigenous communities, FASD was not a dominant lens through which the majority of stories were reported. Rather, it provided a backdrop for discussion about alcohol and pregnancy. The 'blame risk taking mothers' frame was evident in stories reporting on proposed punitive measures and to paint a picture of irresponsible women continuing to drink in the face of public health advice to the contrary. There was little evidence of the 'community responsibility' frame that situates alcohol consumption during pregnancy in a wider social and cultural context. 'Contested evidence and advice' and 'women's rights' were the most prominent frames and in this article we focus on how they were actively deployed to tell the story of alcohol in pregnancy.

Contested evidence and advice

News and popular health stories about alcohol and pregnancy foregrounded 'contested evidence and advice' in three ways: they juxtaposed conflicting expert advice and research findings, highlighted women's 'confusion', and actively promoted opposition to the official guidelines. Newly published scientific research provided a key source of news about the risks associated with alcohol consumption during pregnancy, with stories reporting on studies that variously identified evidence of harm, or no harm, to the fetus from alcohol consumption during pregnancy. Two stories from the *Mother and Baby* website provide an example of the flow of contested evidence. A story headlined 'Light drinking in pregnancy won't harm your child, study suggests' (*Mother and Baby*, 2013a) reported in the lead that:

> Drinking one standard glass of wine a week during pregnancy will not lead to cognitive or behavioural problems in childhood, according to new UK research.

The article drew on the readily available news subsidy provided by the NHMRC to report that the findings go against official guidelines in Australia and elsewhere, which recommend abstinence. In clear contrast, another *Mother and Baby* story, 'Zero alcohol during pregnancy, study says' (*Mother and Baby*, 2013b) reported on the findings of a study about the impact of alcohol on the brain circuitry of mice, including brain and behavioural characteristics similar to those found in FASD. The lead reported that:

> Neuroscientists have found prenatal exposure to alcohol severely disrupts brain development, leading to changes in behaviour such as increased anxiety.

Conflicting evidence and advice also characterized reporting on the issue in mainstream Australian newspapers. For example, a story in *The Australian* headlined 'On balance, no harm in daily tipple for mum' (Smyth, 2013) reported on a Bristol University study showing that moderate drinking (described in the lead as a daily glass of wine) does not cause harm. This headline was countered by expert commentary from Britain's Royal College of Midwives saying that the advice continues to be that it is best for women to avoid alcohol. Just a few months later this newspaper reported in a much more fear-provoking manner that 'pregnant women who drink as little as two glasses of wine in a session could be setting their kids up to fail in school' (Parnell, 2013). It reported on the findings of an Australian study that children of women who frequently drank moderate amounts when pregnant performed less well in school tests by the age of 11.

    Another group of articles drawing on the 'contested evidence' frame did not merely juxtapose contradictory evidence and advice, but positioned women as 'confused' by such contestation. For example, the academic authors of a *Canberra Times* story headlined 'Women still in dark about drinking while pregnant' (Jowsey & Dennis, 2013) cited confusion among their pregnant friends who wondered whether it was okay to have a glass of wine with dinner. The article stated that 'the [NHMRC] Guidelines do not point to any compelling evidence' about the risks of low-level alcohol consumption. The authors argued for more research to provide clarity about questions regarding the critical stages of pregnancy at which point consumption could be harmful and whether a glass of wine at times could be safe. A television news story (*Ten News*, 2014) continued this 'confusion' theme within the 'contested evidence' frame, deriding the medical profession for its failure to provide women with definitive advice about the risks of drinking alcohol while pregnant:

> It's hard to believe these days but there is still confusion over whether or not pregnant women should drink alcohol. We learned today that part of the problem is that many doctors don't even know … mothers say the advice is confusing and inconsistent.

A third set of stories contributing to the 'contested evidence and advice' frame reported on non-medical research that openly challenged the NHMRC abstinence advice. The lead paragraph in *The Daily Telegraph's* 'Pregnant pours' (O'Brien, 2013) story firmly positioned advice from a non-expert on drinking alcohol safely during pregnancy as a contentious one:

> Pregnant women can safely drink two glasses of wine and four cups of coffee a day, according to a controversial new book.

Economist Emily Oster's suggestion that two drinks per day were acceptable was immediately positioned as contradicting official guidelines. In addition to describing the book as 'controversial', the article provided an expert medical opinion opposing the research, referred to the risks of Fetal Alcohol Syndrome (FAS), and quoted from NHMRC Guidelines that there is no safe level of drinking during pregnancy.

    In 2014, the issue of whether the NHMRC Guidelines may themselves be having unintended and unwanted effects received widespread media attention following a letter written by a pharmacist, Ron Batagol, and published in the *Medical Journal of Australia* (see Batagol, 2014). On 21 April 2014 his letter formed the basis of widespread reporting in the mainstream press, with headlines such as:

> Calls to relax pregnancy alcohol guidelines. (Wilson, 2014, p. 7)

> Pharmacist Ron Batagol calls for drinking mothers to be reassured. (Medew, 2014)

These stories reported that Batagol was urging the NHMRC to 'change its alcohol warnings to pregnant women to avoid frightening them into inappropriate terminations'. A television story on *Seven Nightly News* (2014) included the following sound bite from Batagol:

> Women shouldn't seek to have alcohol during pregnancy but my concern is if it does happen they need to be reassured. Small amounts of alcohol exposure in early pregnancy is not a cause for termination.

The reporter referred to statistics showing that 59% of women admitted to drinking while pregnant (cf. AIHW, 2014) by way of introducing a General Practitioner, Dr Ginni Mansberg, who was adamant that the Guidelines are clear and that the last thing women need is reassurance that it is okay to drink. Accommodating the logic of the television format, *Seven News* quoted her stating unequivocally that:

> If anything they need to be told that actually 'no, drinking is not okay in pregnancy'. The Guidelines are black and white and right now with the best evidence available there is no safe level of drinking in pregnancy.

It was noteworthy that the day after Batagol made headlines ABC's *The Pulse* published a story 'Alcohol in pregnancy: why experts say no', which reported that a recent review of the evidence about low to moderate alcohol exposure during pregnancy by Dr Colleen O'Leary 'found no strong research showing harm from low-level drinking, which she defined as one to two standard drinks but less than seven standard drinks a week' (Johnson, 2014). However, the report went on to state that weaknesses in the studies reviewed meant there can be no conclusion that drinking at these levels is safe. Thus, it reported that O'Leary endorsed the Guidelines but also believes the 'over-interpretation of risk leading to comments such as "even one drink can harm your baby", will lead to more harm than good', with potential for women to consider terminating a pregnancy or hiding a drinking habit and avoiding getting help (see also O'Leary & Bower, 2012).

This online report prompted several responses including one from Batagol who took the opportunity to clarify his position and emphasize that he was focusing on the subset of women who may have had intermittent exposure to alcohol before knowing they were pregnant. He offered this argument:

> I believe that it is nothing short of demeaning to this specific group of women, to presume that we can't provide them with the responsible reassurance that they deserve, as is done in various overseas jurisdictions, because we worry about creating a slippery slope mentality for the whole community on the broader question of condoning alcohol exposure during pregnancy.

In the context of this debate it is worth noting that the NHMRC Guidelines do state that the 'risks to the fetus from low-level drinking (such as one or two drinks per week) during pregnancy are likely to be low' (NHMRC, 2009, p. 68), and that 'women who drank alcohol before they knew they were pregnant or during their pregnancy should be reassured that the majority of babies exposed to alcohol suffer no observable harm' (p. 68). Thus, Batagol's comments were largely consistent with the reassurance contained in the Guidelines, while the GP's message was also consistent with the precautionary public health advice. It could also be argued that the unequivocal position she adopted reflects the impetus to restrict public discussion and debate on the issue based on concern for the 'slippery slope mentality' identified in the above comment.

Arguably, what is obscured by this apparent expert disagreement is the distinction the NHMRC Guidelines draw between knowing and unknowing behaviour, whereby the offer of reassurance 'disavows the role of the guidelines in producing this very anxiety' and reinforces the idea that those who knowingly choose to consume some alcohol during pregnancy should not expect or are not worthy of reassurance, even if the scientific evidence base may justify it. They are placed in a different moral category even though their drinking may have occurred at a stage of pregnancy when the fetus is less vulnerable to harm (Keane, 2013, p. 158). This reflects the way in which pronouncements about risks in relation to pregnancy are tied up with social and cultural values and ideas about what it means to be a 'good' or 'bad' mother, as much as they are about science (see Armstrong, 2003).

Alcohol consumption as a woman's right

Against this backdrop of conflicting evidence and advice, we identified a 'women's rights' frame that foregrounded the rights of women to make their own decisions about drinking during pregnancy as well as the right not to be morally judged for their behaviours. Stories adopting this frame tended to emphasize these rights in contrast to interventions that would seek to infringe them. A good example of the clash between these positions was *The Daily Telegraph's* 'Pregnant women warned to adopt zero tolerance approach' (Silmalis, 2013a), which reported in the lead that:

> To drink or not to drink during pregnancy: the age old debate is ramping up with the State Government ordering expectant mothers not to touch a drop of alcohol.

This story referred to a government minister 'instructing' pregnant women to have 'zero tolerance' or 'risk the health of their unborn child' (Silmalis, 2013a). The following day *The Daily Telegraph* published a similar story but opted for a different emphasis with the headline 'Mums raise a glass half full to quiet tipple …' (Silmalis, 2013b), which reported in the lead that:

> A cool, refreshing sip of beer was a major pregnancy craving for Coogee's Jennifer Dean, who gave birth to twins Max and Lily on Tuesday.

It quoted the Sydney mother as saying she did not feel the need to cut the occasional drink out while she was pregnant and she said 'I am happy with my decision. I am not going to put my kids at risk intentionally'. The story then said: 'It might seem like every woman's choice but not according to the NSW Government, which has reiterated its insistence on abstinence'. These stories drew on populist arguments attacking the 'nanny state' mentality of some public health organisations, and openly questioning alcohol guidelines, at the same time drawing on what Keane (2009) has identified as the 'pleasure' discourse of alcohol consumption. This framing worked to position women's freedom to choose as the common sense viewpoint, with government policy as a potential threat to that choice.

In the context of the 'women's rights' frame, consuming alcohol during pregnancy is not constructed primarily as a matter of scientific research or expert opinion but as one of many social practices women negotiate during pregnancy. The issue of women's rights was a common topic in online forums discussing alcohol and pregnancy. For example, some of the typical features of discussions on the *Mommyish* forum included recognition that the majority of mothers have the best interests of their baby at heart; that the science is inconclusive about the risks of moderate consumption; and that it is not helpful for women to be judging each other. Such stories also showed that women do not make their decisions out of ignorance or any wilful desire to harm their babies, or simply in response to a pregnancy craving as mentioned in the above story, but because they do not believe the occasional drink is going to cause harm, which is often based on their personal experience or observations of others and active weighing up of available evidence and advice.

Discussion and conclusions

Our analysis suggests that by framing alcohol consumption during pregnancy in terms of 'contested evidence and advice' and 'women's rights', news and popular health media can be seen as complicating the Australian Government's unequivocal advice. Far from unquestioningly supporting the abstinence message or fuelling the 'FASD crisis' frame, our study found that media reporting highlighted scientific uncertainty and conflicting expert evidence and opinion, providing a corrective to the 'official' abstinence message. This constitutes a challenge to a hierarchical expert-to-lay model of communication wherein journalists assume the role of transferring scientific 'facts' to the lay public in support of a 'correct' public health imperative. Likewise, stories emphasizing 'women's rights' appeared to challenge the biomedical authority model of health communication by privileging women's own voices and knowledge over that of expert authority (see Briggs & Hallin, 2016).

Much media discussion works subtly to question scientific and government attempts to provide an unambiguous message. It was common for reports to juxtapose one set of categorical advice (drinking in moderation is okay) against another set of advice (not drinking is the safest option). This is consistent with previous research showing that news stories often endorse abstinence at the same time as suggesting that low or moderate levels are safe (Bogren, 2011; Rodriguez, 2013). Rodriguez (2013, p. 28) argues: '[t]he message of abstinence is therefore belittled and becomes suggestive rather than assertive, potentially decreasing its authority and influence over the behaviour of expectant mothers'. We would argue, however, that discussion of the issue in news media and popular pregnancy and parenting blogs reflects the inconclusiveness of evidence about the risks of low to moderate consumption and also shows women critically engaging with public health advice in the context of the numerous dos and don'ts they are inundated with during pregnancy (see Lupton, 2012).

News media are often criticized by medical researchers and public health advocates for inaccurate, alarmist or sensational reporting of health and medicine. Such criticisms tend to be tied to certain assumptions about the 'facts' of an issue and who or what is the most authoritative source of knowledge about it. In the case of alcohol during pregnancy, the NHMRC Guidelines are positioned and deployed by journalists and news sources as an authoritative source of knowledge. Thus, any news media departure from the abstinence advice may be criticized as irresponsible and potentially putting expectant mothers and their offspring at risk. However, this approach is grounded in a limited view of the role of news media in reporting on health issues, which fails to acknowledge the mediatization of the health domain (Briggs & Hallin, 2016). Our analyses suggest that reporting is not necessarily a deliberate attempt on the part of irresponsible journalists to distort issues or undermine public health advice. Certainly, news values are a key consideration for journalists, but it is also important to recognize that health and medical sources may incorporate media logics into their own practices such that nuance gives way to alarmist statements of risk.

The letter to the *Medical Journal of Australia* by pharmacist Ron Batagol was arguably deemed newsworthy because of the status of the journal and the fact that he drew attention to the potentially unintended consequences of public health advice. Such expert opinion, along with new research findings, inevitably attracts news media attention and provides stories that journalists perceive as relevant and important to their audiences. Unlike the public health establishment, the role of journalists is not to promote adherence to particular health and medical recommendations but to report that which is deemed newsworthy. This could take the form of providing audiences with a range of information and advice which they are invited to consult in their health decisions. Equally, it may take the form of disrupting lay/professional hierarchies and inviting audiences to observe and judge debate within the medical community (Briggs & Hallin, 2016). These orientations were evident in stories adopting the 'women's rights' and 'contested evidence and advice' frames.

Stories drawing on the 'women's rights' frame tended to emphasize individual women's personal experience of pregnancy and to place responsibility for alcohol consumption with them. The flipside of privileging a woman's individual responsibility is that it could lead to the blaming of mothers for having a child with FASD, without regard for the availability of resources to manage the conception and pregnancy or the constraints of their social circumstances on their choices. Emphasizing responsibility without recognizing limitations on agency perpetuates a neoliberal discourse that eschews the social and cultural context in which women do drink during pregnancy. Thus, it is critical to recognize that the 'women's rights' frame is not simply about emphasizing personal responsibility against government interventions but, rather, it incorporates an appreciation that women's agency in relation to risks and access to resources can often be constrained by their social circumstances. In this context, simply promoting the abstinence message may actually prove counterproductive in that women may not necessarily accept it on face value and in the absence of both convincing scientific evidence and their own situated knowledge and resources. Research also shows that women are sensitive to practices of policing pregnant women and recognize the potential for well-intentioned public health messages to exacerbate women's feelings of guilt and anxiety (Holland et al., 2016; Keane, 2013; Lowe & Lee, 2010; O'Leary & Bower, 2012).

It is not our intention to draw any direct causal relationship between how the issue of alcohol and pregnancy is reported and women's understandings and practices, but we would offer the following concluding observations and suggestions for further consideration. The *Four Corners* programme with which we introduced this article provides a powerful example of the role of this genre of investigative journalism in highlighting issues such as FASD, including the role and responsibility of governments and the medical establishment in taking it seriously and of women as advocates for their children. FASD is clearly a concern for governments, public health advocates and affected families, forming an important dimension of mediated discussion about the consumption of alcohol during pregnancy. It coexists, as we have shown in this article, with news reports and associated commentary on new research findings about the effects of low to moderate alcohol consumption during pregnancy, government calls to action, and women's experiences. The combination of a fracturing and abundant media environment and an increasingly mediatized public health domain challenge a unitary and authoritative public health messaging about drinking during pregnancy. We would argue that media in regard to this issue should be seen and approached by researchers and advocates alike not in terms of its deviation from or adherence to the abstinence advice but for its potential to invite audiences as citizen-consumers to appreciate the complexities, contradictions and uncertainties of scientific evidence, public health advice and lived experiences.

Note

1. 'Hidden Harm' was also the title of the House of Representatives FASD inquiry report, FASD: The Hidden Harm: Inquiry into the prevention, diagnosis and management of FASDs (The Parliament of the Commonwealth of Australia, 2012).

Acknowledgements

We would like to acknowledge Alexandra Walton for her research assistance on the project and Prof. R. Warwick Blood, University of Canberra, for his contributions to the research.

Disclosure statement

No potential conflict of interest was reported by the authors.

Funding

This work is supported by a grant from the Foundation for Alcohol Research and Education (FARE) in Australia. The views presented in this paper are those of the authors.

ORCID

Kerry McCallum ⓘD http://orcid.org/0000-0001-7567-2125
Kate Holland ⓘD http://orcid.org/0000-0003-3873-5769

References

ABC. (2015, November 2). Hidden Harm: Mothers and their children speak up about the devastating legacy of drinking alcohol while pregnant. *Four Corners*. Retrieved from http://www.abc.net.au/4corners/hidden-harm-promo/6896966

AIHW. (2014). *National drug strategy household survey detailed report 2013*. Canberra: AIHW.

Armstrong, E. M. (1998). Diagnosing moral disorder: The discovery and evolution of fetal alcohol syndrome. *Social Science and Medicine, 47*(12), 2025–2042.

Armstrong, E. M. (2003). *Conceiving risk bearing responsibility: Fetal alcohol syndrome and the diagnosis of moral disorder*. Baltimore, MD: The Johns Hopkins University Press.

Batagol, R. P. (2014). Changes in alcohol consumption in pregnant Australian women between 2007 and 2011. *The Medical Journal of Australia, 200*(7), 391–392.

Beck, U. (1992). *Risk society: Towards a new modernity*. London: Sage.

Bell, K., McNaughton, D., & Salmon, A. (2009). Medicine, morality and mothering: Public health discourses on foetal alcohol exposure, smoking around children and childhood overnutrition. *Critical Public Health, 19*(2), 155–170.

Blood, R. W., & Holland, K. (2004). Risky news, madness and public crisis. *Journalism: Theory, Practice & Criticism, 5*(3), 323–342.

Blood, W., Dare, A., McCallum, K., Holland, K., & Pirkis, J. (2008, July 9–11). Enduring and competing news frames: Australian newspaper coverage of the deaths by suicides of two Melbourne girls. In E. Tilley (Ed.), *Power & place: Refereed Proceedings of the Australian & New Zealand Communication Association Conference* (pp. 1–21). Wellington: Massey University.

Bogren, A. (2011). Gender and alcohol: The Swedish press debate. *Journal of Gender Studies, 20*(2), 155–169.

Briggs, C. L., & Hallin, D. (2016). *Making health public: How news coverage is remaking media, medicine and contemporary life.* Abingdon: Routledge.

Callinan, S., & Room, R. (2012). *Alcohol consumption during pregnancy: Results from the 2010 national drug strategy household survey.* Canberra: Centre for Alcohol Policy Research, and the Foundation for Alcohol Research and Education.

Carlisle, S., & Hanlon, P. (2007). Well-being and consumer culture: A different kind of public health problem? *Health Promotion International, 22*(3), 261–268.

CDC. (2016). Alcohol and pregnancy: Why take the risk? Retrieved from http://www.cdc.gov/vitalsigns/fasd/index.html

Colvin, L., Payne, J., Parsons, D., Kurinczuk, J. J., & Bower, C. (2007). Alcohol consumption during pregnancy in nonindigenous West Australian women. *Alcoholism: Clinical and Experimental Research, 31*(2), 276–284.

Couldry, N., & Hepp, A. (2013). Conceptualizing mediatization: Contexts, traditions, arguments. *Communication Theory, 23*(3), 191–202.

D'Angelo, P. (2002). News framing as a multiparadigmatic research program: A response to Entman. *Journal of Communication, 52*(4), 870–888.

Day, K., Gough, B., & McFadden, M. (2004). Warning! Alcohol can seriously damage your feminine health. *Feminist Media Studies, 4*(2), 165–183.

De Vreese, C. (2014). Mediatization of news: The role of journalistic framing. In F. Esser & J. Strombäck (Eds.), *Mediatization of politics* (pp. 137–155). London: Palgrave McMillan.

Donnelly, L. (2015, June 21). Pregnant women should not drink any alcohol BMA warn. *The Telegraph.* Retrieved from http://www.telegraph.co.uk/news/health/news/11689791/Pregnant-women-should-not-drink-any-alcohol-BMA-warn.html

Elliott, E. (2014). Australia plays 'catch-up' with Fetal Alcohol Spectrum Disorders. *The International Journal of Alcohol and Drug Research, 3*(1), 121–125.

Fogarty, A. S., & Chapman, S. (2012). Australian television news coverage of alcohol, health and related policies, 2005 to 2010: Implications for alcohol policy advocates. *Australian & New Zealand Journal of Public Health, 36*(6), 530–536.

Foundation for Alcohol Research and Education. (2016). Retrieved from http://www.fare.org.au

Gamson, W. A., & Modigliani, A. (1989). Media discourse and public opinion on nuclear power: A constructionist approach. *American Journal of Sociology, 95*(1), 1–37.

Gentile, K. (2011). What about the baby? The new cult of domesticity and media images of pregnancy. *Studies in Gender and Sexuality, 12*(1), 38–58.

Hansen, A., & Gunter, B. (2007). Constructing public and political discourse on alcohol issues: Towards a framework for analysis. *Alcohol and Alcoholism, 42*(2), 150–157.

Holmes, B. J. (2009). Media coverage of Canada's obesity epidemic: Illustrating the subtleties of surveillance medicine. *Critical Public Health, 19*(2), 223–233.

Holland, K. (2017). Making mental health news: Australian journalists' views on news values, sources and reporting challenges. *Journalism Studies.* doi:10.1080/1461670X.2017.1304826

Holland, K., McCallum, K., & Blood, R. W. (2015). *Conversations about alcohol and pregnancy.* Canberra: Foundation for Alcohol Research and Education.

Holland, K., McCallum, K., & Walton, A. (2016). 'I'm not clear on what the risk is': Women's reflexive negotiations of uncertainty about alcohol during pregnancy. *Health, Risk and Society, 18*(1–2), 38–58.

Hunting, G., & Browne, A. J. (2012). Decolonizing policy discourse: Reframing the 'problem' of fetal alcohol spectrum disorder. *Women's Health and Urban Life, 11*(1), 35–53.

Johnson, C. (2014, April 22). Alcohol in pregnancy: Why experts say no. *ABC Pulse.* Retrieved from http://www.abc.net.au/health

Jowsey, T., & Dennis, S. (2013, October 10). Women still in dark about drinking while pregnant. *The Canberra Times,* B004.

Keane, H. (2009). Intoxication, harm and pleasure: An analysis of the Australian National Alcohol Strategy. *Critical Public Health, 19*(2), 135–142.

Keane, H. (2013). Healthy adults and maternal bodies: Reformulations of gender in Australian alcohol guidelines. *Health Sociology Review, 22*(2), 151–161.

Leask, J., Hooker, C., & King, C. (2010). Media coverage of health issues and how to work more effectively with journalists: A qualitative study. *BMC Public Health, 10,* 535–541.

Leppo, A. (2012). The emergence of the foetus: Discourses on foetal alcohol syndrome prevention and compulsory treatment in Finland. *Critical Public Health, 22*(2), 179–191.

Lowe, P. K., & Lee, E. J. (2010). Advocating alcohol abstinence to pregnant women: Some observations about British policy. *Health, Risk and Society, 12*(4), 301–311.

Lupton, D. (2011). 'The best thing for the baby': Mothers' concepts and experiences related to promoting their infants' health and development. *Health, Risk and Society, 13*(7–8), 637–651.

Lupton, D. (2012). 'Precious cargo': Foetal subjects, risk and reproductive citizenship. *Critical Public Health, 22*(3), 329–340.

Lupton, D. (2013). *The social worlds of the unborn*. Basingstoke: Palgrave Macmillan.

Lyerly, A. D., Mitchell, L. M., Armstrong, E. M., Harris, L. H., Kukla, R., Kuppermann, M., & Little, M. O. (2009, November–December). Risk and the pregnant body. *Hastings Center Report, 39*(6), 34–42.

McCallum, K. & Waller, L. (2017). The dimensions of mediatized policy-making in Australian Indigenous affairs. *Communications: The European Journal of Communication, 42*(2), 173–193.

Medew, J. (2014, April 21). Pharmacist Ron Batagol calls for drinking mothers to be reassured. *Sydney Morning Herald*. Retrieved from http://www.smh.com.au/national/pharmacist-ron-batagol-calls-for-drinking-mothers-to-be-reassured-20140420-36ytp.html

Mother and Baby. (2013a, April 18). Light drinking in pregnancy won't harm your child, study suggests. Retrieved from http://www.motherandbaby.com.au

Mother and Baby. (2013b, December 5). Zero alcohol during pregnancy, study says.... Retrieved from http://www.motherandbaby.com.au

NHMRC. (2009). *Guidelines to reduce health risks from drinking alcohol*. Canberra: Commonwealth of Australia.

O'Brien, S. (2013, August 16). Pregnant pours. *The Daily Telegraph*, p. 3.

O'Leary, C. M., & Bower, C. (2012). Guidelines for pregnancy: What's an acceptable risk, and how is the evidence (finally) shaping up? *Drug and Alcohol Review, 31*, 170–183.

Parnell, S. (2013, October 16). Health. *The Australian*, p. 14.

Peadon, E., Payne, J., Henley, N., D'Antoine, H., Bartu, A., O'Leary, C., ... Elliott, E. J. (2011). Attitudes and behaviour predict women's intention to drink alcohol during pregnancy: The challenge for health professionals. *BMC Public Heath, 11*, 584.

Powers, J. R., Loxton, D. J., Burns, L. A., Shakeshaft, A., Elliott, E. J., & Dunlop, A. J. (2010). Assessing pregnant women's compliance with different alcohol guidelines: An 11-year prospective study. *Medical Journal of Australia, 192*(12), 690–693.

Rail, G., & Beausoleil, N. (2003). Introduction to "Health Panic and Women's Health". *Atlantis: Critical Studies in Gender, Culture & Social Justice, 27*(2), 1–5.

Reese, S. (2007). The framing project: A bridging model for media research revisited. *Journal of Communication, 57*, 148–154.

Rodriguez, I. E. (2013). *Analysis of media portrayal of alcohol consumption during pregnancy and Fetal Alcohol Spectrum Disorder (FASD) in Australian print media*. Canberra: Foundation for Alcohol Research and Education.

Seven Nightly News. (2014, April 21). Alcohol review: A leading pharmacist is calling for alcohol warnings for pregnant women to be reviewed and relaxed.

Shugart, H. A. (2011). Heavy viewing: Emergent frames in contemporary news coverage of obesity. *Health Communication, 26*(7), 635–648.

Silmalis, L. (2013a, September 7). Pregnant women warned to adopt zero tolerance approach to alcohol intake. *The Daily Telegraph*. Retrieved from http://www.dailytelegraph.com.au

Silmalis, L. (2013b, September 8). Mums raise a glass half full to quiet tipple. *The Daily Telegraph*, p. 31.

Smyth, C. (2013, June 19). On balance, no harm in daily tipple for mum. *The Australian*, p. 3.

Ten News. (2014, July 1). It's hard to believe these days but there are still confusion over whether or not pregnant women should drink alcohol.

The Parliament of the Commonwealth of Australia. (2012, November). FASD: The hidden harm. Inquiry into the prevention, diagnosis and management of fetal alcohol spectrum disorders. *House of Representatives. Standing Committee on Social Policy and Legal Affairs*.

Turner, G. (2016). *Re-inventing media*. London: Routledge.

Van Gorp, B. (2007). The constructionist approach to framing: Bringing culture back in. *Journal of Communication, 57*, 60–78.

Watkins, J., Park, S., Blood, W., Deas, M., Dunne Breen, M., Fisher, C., ... Ricketson, M. (2016). *Digital news report: Australia 2016*. Canberra: News & Media Research Centre.

Wilson, L. (2014, April 21). Calls to relax pregnancy alcohol guidelines. *The Daily Telegraph*, 7.

5   Working up a lather

The rise (and fall?) of hand hygiene in
Canadian newspapers, 1986–2015

Emma Whelan

ABSTRACT

Hand hygiene is a long-standing concern in the health sciences literature, but its emergence as a public health issue in the news is a more recent development. Drawing on Alan Hunt's work on moral regulation and responsibilization, this article analyses 30 years of Canadian newspaper coverage of hand hygiene. Concerns associated with hand hygiene and trends in coverage were identified in a sample of 518 articles, published between 1986 and 2015. Although the Severe Acute Respiratory Syndrome (SARS) and H1N1 influenza epidemics emerged as important triggers, healthcare-associated infection (HAI) was the dominant trigger for hand hygiene coverage. The articles tend to present hand hygiene as a unidimensional approach to infection control. They tend to responsibilize individuals–first members of the general public, then healthcare providers and increasingly patients–for managing the risk of infection, rather than focus upon social, cultural, political and economic factors that would promote a more broad-based and structural response to HAI.

Introduction

The link between handwashing and the prevention of infectious disease was made in the early nineteenth century (Boyce & Pittet, 2002); the discovery is often attributed to Hungarian obstetrician Ignaz Semmelweis (Bjerke, 2004). While Semmelweis's findings initially had little impact, the late nineteenth century brought growing acceptance with Pasteur's germ theory and Lister's work on antisepsis (Gillies, 2005). Medline, the US National Library of Medicine's database, indexes journal articles as far back as 1921 (Conover & Laird, 1921) that advocate better disinfection of the hands. Thus, handwashing is an issue of long-standing importance in the medical literature. But only more recently has 'hand hygiene' (now the usual term, which includes the use of hand sanitizer) become a focal public health concern. Discussions about hand hygiene now extend beyond the health sciences and attempt to engage the public. This is reflected in an expansion of news coverage of handwashing as a public health issue.

While news coverage does not straightforwardly determine public perceptions of health issues, it plays a key role in cultural preoccupation with health matters, and has an agenda-setting effect in public health (Barnes et al., 2008; Holmes, 2009; Kim, Kumanyika, Shive, Igweatu, & Kim, 2010; Zhang, Jin, Stewart, & Porter, 2016). Rather than reflecting reality transparently, news media 'filter and shape it' (Barnes et al., 2008, p. 605), focusing on some health issues and not others, influencing public perceptions of their relative importance, and thereby affecting the development of public health policies.

Supplemental data for this article can be accessed here. [https://doi.org/10.1080/09581596.2018.1453126]

The news media's framing of issues moulds understandings of social problems by identifying causes, endorsing solutions, urging public support and making moral assessments (Kim et al., 2010). Discussions in the news of who is responsible for causing and solving health problems 'may exert an indirect yet significant influence on health policies and practices regarding societal resource allocations in the prevention, intervention and treatment efforts of public health problems' (Zhang et al., 2016, p. 119). Research suggests that when news coverage of issues focuses on individuals or groups, the public is more likely to blame those individuals or groups for the issues, whereas framing issues as societal problems tends to influence the public to hold governmental agencies responsible (Kim et al., 2010). Thus, how hand hygiene is covered in the news media affects public perceptions and, ultimately, public health policy – including how responsibility for hand hygiene is apportioned.

Using the concepts of moral regulation and responsibilization (Hunt, 1999, 2003), this article examines Canadian newspapers' coverage of hand hygiene from 1986 to 2015, with a focus on how coverage frames responsibility for preventing infectious disease. While epidemic diseases in the community, like Severe Acute Respiratory Syndrome (SARS) and the H1N1 influenza virus, were prominent triggers of Canadian news coverage of hand hygiene, reporting on healthcare-associated infection (HAI)[1] accounts for the greatest proportion of coverage, particularly in later years. Relatedly, responsibility for hand hygiene shifted over time, from a focus on public handwashing to curb the spread of disease in the community, to the responsibility of healthcare providers to clean their hands to prevent healthcare-associated infection (HAI). However, the last few years of coverage show a growing tendency to responsibilize patients for ensuring *healthcare providers'* good hand hygiene. I conclude with a discussion of the Canadian news media's contributions to a model of hand hygiene as the primary method of infection prevention, one that focuses on individual behaviour and education and deemphasizes power dynamics and structural dimensions of infectious disease transmission. This article thereby contributes to critiques of public health's focus on individual choices and behaviours in addressing health problems, and of its relative neglect of social causes of, and solutions to, health problems (Ayo, 2012; Lindsay, 2010; Raphael, 2008; Thompson & Kumar, 2011).

Hand hygiene and the social sciences

Critical analyses of hand hygiene are rare in the social sciences. A recent wave of historical and social scientific works focus on cleanliness as a social, political and cultural issue (Bashford, 2004; Brown, 2011; Burnstein, 2006; Campkin & Cox, 2013; Hoy, 1995; Kelley, 2010; Smith, 2007; Stow, 2012; Vigarello, 2008), but these works say surprisingly little about hand hygiene. Social scientists have helped to *promote* hand hygiene by exploring 'barriers' to, and programs that may encourage, good hand hygiene (e.g. Aunger et al., 2010; Contzen, Meili, & Mosler, 2015; Curtis et al., 2003; London School of Hygiene & Tropical Medicine, 2000; VanSteelandt, Conly, Ghali, & Mather, 2015; Wilson, Jacob, & Powell, 2011). Such literature is more focused on improving compliance with hand hygiene campaigns than on analysing them, though some of it analyses the effects of sociocultural factors on compliance (see Wilson et al., 2011). There is a small critical literature on hand hygiene campaigns in developing countries; Bexell (2013) and Plyushteva (2009), for instance, provide essential critiques of the Global Public–Private Partnership for Handwashing with Soap (PPP-HW). According to Plyushteva (2009), this top-down initiative reflects the interests of the three main multinational soap companies, Unilever, Proctor & Gamble and Colgate-Palmolive, depicting people in the Global South as ignorant of the facts of hygiene and as ripe targets for market expansion. It does little to address the effects of structural inequality in impoverished communities, like lack of access to clean water and sewage management systems, that often make handwashing with soap a moot point (Plyushteva, 2009; see also Langford & Panter-Brick, 2013). Hand hygiene campaigns in wealthy countries have largely escaped critical scrutiny, however.

This article builds on critical analyses of hygiene-focused approaches to infection control, and of coverage of antibiotic-resistant 'superbugs' and infectious disease epidemics in the news media, which discuss hand hygiene as a related issue (Brown, Crawford, Nerlich, & Koteyko, 2008; Brown, Nerlich, Crawford, Koteyko, & Carter, 2009; Crawford & Brown, 2008; Koteyko, Nerlich, Crawford, & Wright, 2008;

Nerlich, 2009; Washer & Joffe, 2006). For instance, Koteyko et al. (2008) argue that 'proper' hand hygiene is often represented, both in the UK news media and by diverse parties in healthcare and politics, as a 'simple' solution to superbugs: 'Presenting MRSA [Methicillin-resistant *Staphylococcus aureus*] as a problem amenable to simple solutions, such as cleanliness, handwashing, or the abolition of NHS targets, works as a reassurance that things are, or will be, under control' (p. 238). They note that the media's almost exclusive focus on cleanliness in hospitals occludes other approaches to managing MRSA, such as screening and isolation (Koteyko et al., 2008). My research provides further support for such arguments. However, to my knowledge, the present article is the first to focus specifically on hand hygiene as a news issue, and on how responsibility for hand hygiene is presented in news coverage.

Canadian public health and hand hygiene

This study developed out of my curiosity about a marked increase in the 2000s of information about hand hygiene directed at Canadian adults, including the growing presence of handwashing posters and guidelines in public restrooms and Canadian newspaper articles promoting hand hygiene. To gauge whether this new focus on handwashing was specific to Canada, I and a research assistant conducted an exploratory search of the LexisNexis News database in 2013, using the Major Newspapers search function. This international English language newspapers data-set is dominated by American, Australian and British papers; it includes only three Canadian newspapers, yet all three placed in the top five papers for coverage of handwashing.[2] Thus, Canada seems to be a hotbed of hand hygiene coverage. This article reports on the next stage of the research, which explored how and why hand hygiene was represented as an important public health issue in Canadian newspapers.

Two recent Canadian public health issues help to make sense of the rise of hand hygiene coverage in Canada. First, the SARS epidemic of 2003 affected Canada (particularly Toronto) and several Asian countries far more significantly than other countries. In the absence of effective prophylactics for SARS, traditional infection prevention methods were used to contain its spread, and handwashing was particularly promoted (National Advisory Committee on SARS & Public Health, 2003; Nicolle, 2007; Ofner, Lem, Sarwal, Vearncombe, & Simor, 2003; Parini, 2003). Critics of Canada's management of the crisis pointed to the inadequacies of the country's public health and infection control systems, including a lack of funding, training, leadership and coordination[3] (Mowat & Butler-Jones, 2007; National Advisory Committee on SARS & Public Health, 2003; Ontario Agency for Health Protection & Promotion, & Provincial Infectious Diseases Advisory Committee, 2012). The crisis became the impetus for changes in the public health infrastructure, such as the founding in 2004 of the Public Health Agency of Canada, which has spearheaded many initiatives on infectious diseases, with a strong focus on hand hygiene (Federal/Provincial/Territorial Special Task Force on Public Health, 2005; Mowat & Butler-Jones, 2007; Stachenko, Legowski, & Geneau, 2009).

Second, healthcare-associated infection is a prominent concern in Canada. The Canadian Nosocomial Infection Surveillance Program was initiated in 1994 to gather data and establish benchmarks and guidelines for Canadian hospitals (http://www.phac-aspc.gc.ca/nois-sinp/survprog-eng.php). The SARS crisis had a major impact on infection control practices in Canadian hospitals (Butler-Jones, 2013), and Canada has been an enthusiastic participant in the World Health Organization's (WHO) 'Clean Care is Safer Care' initiative, begun in 2005 to reduce HAI primarily through hand hygiene (WHO, 2011, p. 24). Yet despite these efforts, Canada's HAI prevalence rate ranks second only to New Zealand among high income countries (WHO, 2011, p. 13). Restructuring/defunding of the healthcare system is said to have increased HAI due to reductions in healthcare staff, increased patient-provider ratios and inadequately resourced infection control in healthcare facilities (Nosocomial & Occupational Infections Section, 2010). Concerns about inadequate reporting and monitoring of HAI within healthcare facilities and across levels of government persist (Blackwell, 2015; McCarter, 2008; Silversides, 2009). But while structural issues have been linked to the persistent problem of HAI, good personal hand hygiene is often promoted as the primary solution by the Canadian public health establishment (e.g. Butler-Jones, 2013).

As Raphael (2008) has pointed out, a structural approach to public health has long been marginalized in Canada, where health policy typically focuses on individual lifestyles and healthy choices. Although it is widely acknowledged that the problems of SARS and HAI are connected to *structural* problems in Canada's hospitals and public health system, by triggering such an intense focus on hand hygiene, these epidemics paradoxically seem to have increased the focus on *individual* choices, behaviours and responsibilities as solutions to Canadian public health problems.

Responsibilization

I address the question of responsibility for health using a framework derived from the work of Hunt (1999, 2003) on moral regulation. The identification of a social problem is usually accompanied by claims about who is responsible for addressing it. To understand attributions of blame and the moral aspects of handwashing campaigns, I consider Hunt's formulation of moral regulation projects as efforts directed not at broader structural or institutional change, but rather at changing 'the conduct and ethical subjectivity of individuals' (Hunt, 1999, p. 17). Such projects often involve responsibilization, a discursive practice by which both self and others are exhorted to act responsibly. Responsibilization 'captures the duality of responsibility for the self and for others by drawing attention to the active components of many discourses that assign responsibility to specific categories of agents as is exemplified in the slogan: "Only you can stop drinking and driving," which individualizes the responsible driver' (Hunt, 1999, p. 223). Similarly, 'Ottawa's health is in your hands', the headline of a hand hygiene poster issued by the Canadian capital city's public health authority (Ottawa Public Health, 2009), individualizes the responsible citizen to wash. In such campaigns, *effects* may be felt at the social or community level, but *action* must be taken by individuals; the responsibility of institutions and organizations and the influence of structural factors beyond individual control are deemphasized. In the case of hand hygiene, institutional responsibility often takes the form of issuing guidelines about behaviour, which individuals may or may not follow.

Hunt points out that 'Increasingly, morality has come to function through proxies, not in its own voice, but in and through other discursive forms, the two most important and closely related being the discourses of "harm" and "risk"' (Hunt, 2003, p. 166). Discourses of harm and risk typically are grounded in scientific authority, obscuring their moral elements by invoking evidence and rational goals. For example, as Koteyko et al. (2008) argue, handwashing is often presented as the 'common sense' solution in government and news discourses about infectious disease risk, based on selective appropriation of scientific evidence that supports this position (and exclusion or ignorance of evidence that does not). The position that you *should* wash your hands (a moral argument) becomes subsumed in the goal of reducing infection; hand-washing is now routinely presented as the obvious, easy way to meet this goal. This mixing of the moral and the utilitarian creates, Hunt argues, a hybrid form of discourse, 'an apparently benign form of moralization in which the boundary between objective hazards and normative judgments becomes blurred' (2003, p. 166–167).

Like many responsibilization projects, hand hygiene campaigns represent methods of 'governing at a distance' that entail both freedom and manipulation (Juhila, Raitakari, & Löfstrand, 2017). Individuals may, on the face of it, choose voluntarily to clean their hands as the guidelines direct, as an act of good citizenship. On the other hand, as Miller and Rose (2008) argue, responsibilized subjects 'have to make decisions about their self-conduct surrounded by a web of vocabularies, injunctions, promises, dire warnings and threats of intervention, organized increasingly around a proliferation of norms and normativities' (p. 205). Within a hybrid moral-scientific discourse, such rules of good citizenship set limits on freedom of choice, and those found not to comply may be blamed (Juhila et al., 2017). In public health, many issues have been individualized to such an extent that 'individuals rather than governments or business are now responsible for managing individual harms and risks' (Ayo, 2012; Lindsay, 2010, p. 481). The media is complicit in this, promoting a bias toward 'individual level explanations' which partly explains the popular tendency to 'prioritize individual responsibility for health problems' (Kim et al., 2010, p. S230). The result is a form of health promotion that focuses on individual choices and behaviours versus the social conditions that influence, and indeed make possible (or impossible), individual choices and behaviours (Raphael, 2008; Thompson & Kumar, 2011).

Methods

To ascertain how handwashing is represented in Canadian newspapers, I conducted searches in the full-text LexisNexis Academic database, using the search terms handwashing (one word), hand washing (two words) and hand hygiene in article headlines and lead paragraphs, restricting results to English-language Canadian newspapers. Searches were completed in the summer of 2016. Search dates were left open to determine when coverage in the database started, but only articles up to the end of 2015 were included in the sample.

Results were screened for relevance to handwashing as a hygiene concern, and duplicate articles (with identical titles, published on the same date in different editions of a newspaper) were deleted. The final sample was 518 articles from 50 newspapers, representing 10 of Canada's 13 provinces and territories. It included articles in papers published in the nation's six largest urban areas, as well as in smaller cities and towns. Canada's most populous province, Ontario, is particularly well-represented; Quebec, the second most populous province, is underrepresented because most Quebecois papers are published in French. The earliest relevant article archived in LexisNexis was published in January 1986, and the latest article in April 2015, with almost 92% of the articles published in 2000 or later. Many of the 50 newspapers represented in the sample are not archived in LexisNexis for the full period of 1986–2015. That said, the fact that 92% of the articles appeared after 2000 seems to be less an artefact of LexisNexis' archiving than the result of a shift toward greater coverage of hand hygiene in many newspapers in the 2000s. See Supplementary Table for the top 15 newspapers in the database, representing 77% of the sample. The nine top papers were archived in LexisNexis well before 2000, but the majority of their hand hygiene articles were published from 2000 on.

A detailed analysis of the sample was conducted to establish which aspects of hand hygiene were most discussed in Canadian papers. In each of the 518 articles, I identified triggers, defined as: issues or concerns presented as important in the headline and opening sentences of the article, such as healthcare providers' poor hand hygiene; the apparent goal of the article, such as education about handwashing technique; and 'news pegs' (Greenberg, Sachsman, Sandman, & Salomone, 1989, p. 120), events presented as rationales for the article's publication, such as the publication of a study about handwashing or a *Clostridium difficile* (*C. difficile*) outbreak in a hospital. I also coded the articles for other concerns not explicitly presented as triggers. The position taken by the article about hand hygiene or hand hygiene campaigns (positive/promotion; negative/critiques; ambivalent/both promotion and critique; or no position), and the type of article (news report; letter; column, usually a physician's column; editorial) also were recorded. Initially, I coded 236 articles to generate a comprehensive list of trigger and other concerns, and then I used this list to (re)code the entire sample of 518 articles (including the original 236) to ensure consistency.

Results

Of the 518 articles analysed, 57 were letters to the editor, 23 were editorials and 18 were columns, usually physicians' columns. The remaining 420, 82% of the sample, were news reports. Thus, most articles to which I refer are news reports; the exceptions are noted as columns, editorials or letters to the editor in the References.

Figure 1 shows that there were peaks in coverage in 2003, the year of the SARS epidemic, and in 2009, the year of the H1N1 epidemic. However, coverage also increased markedly a few years after SARS, two years before the H1N1 scare. Although one might expect the H1N1 crisis of 2009 to boost coverage of hand hygiene, it declines steadily after that, with only two articles published in 2015. Contrary to expectations, the SARS and H1N1 epidemics, while important, provide limited explanation of the

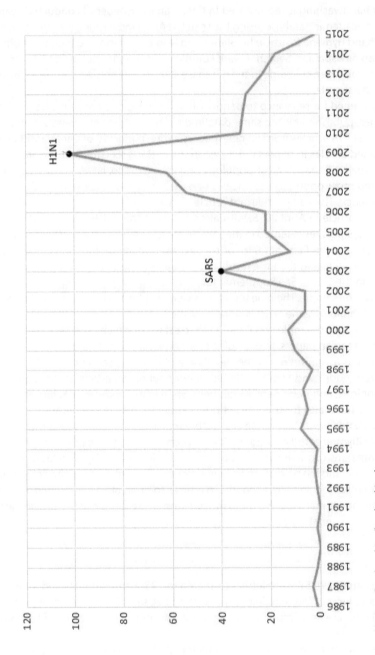

Figure 1. Articles on hand hygiene/hand washing/handwashing by year.

patterns over time. The top triggers and other concerns identified in the sample are listed in Table 1. Many articles had more than one trigger; most mentioned several other concerns as well.

Healthcare providers' hand hygiene and public hand hygiene were both discussed frequently in the sample, as triggers and as mentioned concerns. Public hand hygiene articles tended to present education of the public/readership as a rationale for their publication; some articles even provide explicit 'how-to' handwashing advice, especially during the SARS and the H1N1 scares. By contrast, education of healthcare providers was a trigger relatively rarely, though it was mentioned frequently.

Articles on disease outbreaks, or fears of them, were common. Up until 2006, most focused on the importance of public handwashing to curb infectious disease in the community, particularly SARS and influenza; even articles about outbreaks in hospitals urged visiting members of the public to wash their hands. From 2006 to 2008, the focus begins to shift toward outbreaks in hospitals and healthcare provider hand hygiene, though the H1N1 outbreak in 2009 turns attention temporarily back to the community. By 2010, the focus is decisively on concern about outbreaks in hospitals, particularly *C. difficile*, noroviruses and antibiotic-resistant infections like Vancomycin-Resistant Enterococcus (VRE) and MRSA. Even more common were articles triggered by HAI as a general concept (as opposed to specific diseases), and these focused on healthcare provider hand hygiene. A typical example comes from a *Globe & Mail* report:

> Soaping up or squirting on hand sanitizer seems so simple, but studies show that less than half of hospital nurses and physicians clean their hands between patients. And the results can be deadly: Hospital infections kill 8,000 to 12,000 people a year, according to Health Canada. (Dube, 2007, p. L1)

The timing of this concern is curious. Only 15% of HAI-triggered articles were published before SARS, and despite the intense concern about SARS transmission in hospitals in 2003, only one article discussed HAI as a trigger concern that year. But HAI became a common trigger concern in 2004 and was a trigger for the majority of articles in 2007 and 2008. It is not clear what specifically triggered concerns about HAI in these years. One factor may be the Canadian federal government's 2006 pledge to support the WHO's 'Clean Care is Safer Care' HAI-reduction strategy, based primarily on hand hygiene (http://www. who.int/patientsafety/events/06/gpsc.canada/en/). HAI becomes relatively less important in 2009, the year of the H1N1 outbreak, triggering only 19% of the articles. It becomes dominant again in 2011 (65%), and then declines to 22% by 2014.

Nevertheless, much coverage in later years discusses hospital infection control measures (especially hand hygiene). This suggests that concern about HAI had infiltrated the public consciousness to such

Table 1. Common triggers and other concerns.

Concern/issue/event	Number of articles		
	Trigger	Other concern	TOTAL
Public hand hygiene	181	76	257
HAI in general	175	28	203
Hand hygiene education	161	143	304
Studies or reports published	155	35	190
Healthcare provider hand hygiene	154	66	220
Actual disease outbreak	151	21	172
Specific diseases – fears of outbreak, actual outbreak or approaching season (e.g. flu season)			
Influenza	62	84	146
H1N1	53	10	63
SARS	30	14	44
C. Diff.	25	63	88
Norovirus	25	20	45
Cold	21	54	75
MRSA	3	54	57
VRE	0	19	19
Hand hygiene promotion campaigns	56	40	96
Hand hygiene audit in health care facilities	57	34	91
Cleaning in health care facilities	8	82	90

an extent that the association between HAI and poor hand hygiene no longer needed to be made explicit. For example, three news reports in 2014 address a Canadian study of how monitoring affects hand hygiene compliance among healthcare providers. HAI is mentioned only in passing toward the end of two of the reports; in the third report the only suggestion that concern about HAI motivated this study is the job title of one of the study's co-authors, a medical director of infection prevention and control (O'Connor, 2014, A4). The articles no longer point out the threat of HAI posed by poor hand hygiene; the threat is assumed.

The targets of hand hygiene advice, and the actors responsible for hand hygiene, shift over the 30-year period. In the earlier years, the public was the focus. Articles on studies of public handwashing and on how to wash were common in the 90s and early 2000s. Articles often featured moralizing headlines emphasizing individual responsibility and good citizenship: 'Hand washing – it's the right thing to do' (Gifford-Jones, 1995); 'School children should learn importance of hand-washing' (Knight Ridder Newspapers, 1998). But in 2007, there was a decisive shift toward studies of healthcare workers' hand hygiene. The language about *how* to increase handwashing also shifts, from an early focus on public education, to a later one on compliance rates and auditing of healthcare providers, as hospital monitoring programs become a stronger focus. Thus, Canadian news coverage of handwashing shifted from a health education project directed at the general public and often initiated by the healthcare establishment, to an indictment of healthcare providers' poor hand hygiene. The responsibilization of the public that initially came from the healthcare establishment gets redirected back upon healthcare providers.

That said, the sample did contain several articles, appearing first in 2005 but especially from 2008 on, that discuss the enrolment of patients into healthcare hygiene initiatives. These were not just about getting patients to wash their hands. Fifteen articles, for instance, promote campaigns to encourage patients to *ask their healthcare providers* to wash their hands. A shift in responsibilization occurs, from individual members of the public to individual healthcare providers and, increasingly, the limited success of hospitals' and health authorities' efforts to police healthcare providers is discussed. Health authorities seem to be responding by responsibilizing patients, not just to wash their own hands, but to help solve the problem of their *caregivers'* poor hand hygiene (although a few of these articles admit that patients may feel uncomfortable confronting their healthcare providers):

> [Alberta Health Services chief executive Vickie Kaminski] said Alberta Health Services has embarked on an educational campaign for health-care staff and has installed more hand-washing stations and alcohol-based hand sanitizers in hopes of improving hand hygiene rates. But if patients are concerned, they shouldn't hesitate to ask their nurse or doctor if they have washed their hands, she added. 'A lot of people are uncomfortable with that and they're afraid it might complicate their care, but in actual fact, I think … it reminds the staff member,' she said. 'They don't want to cause you to have an infection and have to stay longer'. (Ibrahim, 2014, p. A3)

As to the position of the articles, only two per cent contained no discernible position on handwashing. The vast majority – 82% – promoted hand hygiene without offering any critical commentary, and often contained strong moral messages. Almost 5% of the sample presented a negative assessment of handwashing or, more often, handwashing campaigns; 11% presented an ambivalent position, discussing handwashing as positive in some respects, but also presenting critiques of handwashing or campaigns. The critical and ambivalent segment of the sample contained proportionally more letters and editorials than the pro-handwashing segment; that said, most reader letters (63%) and editorials (77%) contained only positive messages.

There were no articles presenting ambivalent or critical messages about hand hygiene in the first few years of the sample (1986–1994), and such articles were uncommon in 2003–2006, the year of SARS and its aftermath. Critical comments about handwashing from 1995 to 2002 tended to trivialize hand hygiene, suggesting the concern is overblown. Such pieces sometimes joked about Lady Macbeth and germophobia, but often contained pro-washing messages as well, representing the focus on hand hygiene as relatively harmless, albeit pathetic, excessive or mundane.

> I am careful about germs. Too careful, some might have said – until this week. Until National Handwashing Awareness Week justified every obsessive bit of caution I have ever shown about germs … Despite all my efforts, I remain

vulnerable to the habits of the rest of you, which is why I cheer National Handwashing Awareness Week. (Hughes, 1995, p. B3).

Are we so completely devoid of national confidence that a story about Canadians' vast superiority over the U.S. in hand washing gets front-page coverage? ... It seems that not many days go by where we can't help but compare ourselves to the Americans and scream victory in such B-grade categories as hand washing. (Raymer, 2000, p. A16)

However, critical messages became more frequent and serious when, due to growing concern about HAI, hand hygiene in healthcare comes under fire. A few pieces questioned how effective hand hygiene actually is: 'Sudsing up may not stem spread of flu; Contentious study dismisses preventive benefit of vigorous handwashing' (Vancouver Sun/Canwest News Service, 2009, p. A5). Others critiqued the persistent failure of healthcare hand hygiene campaigns to improve compliance rates long-term, the high costs of such campaigns and their promotion of simplistic information that healthcare providers already know:

Your mother always told you to wash your hands, but I bet she never tried to charge you $16 million for the advice. The province will spend that astonishing amount to promote 'hand hygiene.' Hand washing, to you. Most amazing of all, the recipients of this advice will be the province's many thousands of health-care employees ... Asked what all that money would buy, Health Minister Dave Hancock shrugged, sort of, and said, 'sinks.' And you thought Alberta hospitals had running water ... Hancock is trying to create a central reporting and control system to make sure stringent, uniform standards are applied. The goal is laudable, but for most Albertans, well or ill, it will seem patently absurd that a modern health system has to be taught about hand-washing. (Braid, 2008, p. A4)

Not only does this article ridicule the cost of hand hygiene education, but also Hancock's improvement of handwashing facilities and reporting system in hospitals – structural interventions. The message here is that, if healthcare workers just washed their hands, that would fix the problem, free of charge.

Many articles – both critical/ambivalent and pro-handwashing–targeted healthcare workers for their failure to wash when they should know better: 'All doctors should be cleaning their hands before and after seeing any patient', said B.C. Medical Association president Dr Nasir Jetha. 'Many of us do, but many more don't. There's no excuse for that. As senior medical professionals, doctors should be setting an example' (Baron, 2011, p. A4). There were also a few cases of one professional group (registered nurses) attacking another – sometimes physicians or, as in this letter to the editor, nurse's aides – suggesting that hand hygiene compliance campaigns in the hospitals may be fuelling interprofessional contests amid funding cutbacks:

One vital part missing from Alberta Health Services compliance rates is specifically 'who' is not washing their hands. The article cites nurses and doctors, but does not address nonregulated health-care professionals. Over the past five years, RNs have slowly been replaced in the hospital setting by nurse's aides (NAs). Research has consistently revealed that maintaining more registered nurses in hospital settings leads to improved patient outcomes, a decrease in hospital-associated infections and reduced costs to hospitals. However, *government policy in Alberta has consistently reflected the approach of reducing the number of RNs to cut hospital expenses.* (Vihos, 2014, p. A25; emphasis added)

Others took a structural approach further, discussing the inadequacy of handwashing alone in fighting HAIs in hospitals, and pointing to the neglect of problems like overcrowding, inappropriate use of gloves, inadequate cleaning and outdated facilities. While such messages appeared occasionally before, from 2007 on they become more common and are confined less to reader letters, as in this report:

Hospitals have contracted out cleaning jobs to the lowest bidder in an effort to save money while Ontario residents are lectured on how to promote proper hand washing, unionized health-care workers charge. Thousands of patients will get a hospital-borne infection in Ontario this year like *C. difficile* ... 'So we have to wash our hands, but we don't have to make sure the people washing down beds, rooms, hallways and equipment are part of a system?' [MPP for Hamilton Centre Andrea] Horwath said (Talaga, 2008, p. A23).

But again, critiques of the individual hand hygiene narrative represent a very small minority of news coverage, and are dismissed in other articles:

'If I had a nickel for everybody who said to me that we could fix infections in hospitals if we cleaned elevator buttons I would be a rich woman – the elevator buttons are not the problem,' [infectious disease specialist Dr. Alison] McGeer explained ... 'If you wash your hands regularly, if you don't touch your mouth with your hands, that's much more important than worrying about cleaning the environment.' (Oliveira, 2012, p. A25)

Here, not only is the solution to HAI reduced to cleanliness (Koteyko et al., 2008), but to a specific form of cleanliness: *only* hand hygiene will work.

Discussion

This sample suggests a shift in Canadian news coverage over 30 years, from advocating public hand-washing to curb epidemics, to healthcare providers' responsibility for hand hygiene and HAI. However, recently public responsibility has made a comeback, as patients are increasingly responsibilized for healthcare providers' hand hygiene. A discussion of why HAI became a concern in the news when it did, when HAI rates had been increasing for years, and how coverage of HAI in general changes over time, is beyond the scope of this paper. However, I conclude with some observations about how a hand hygiene focus frames the issues of infection and responsibility in particular ways.

A range of concerned parties, from unions (Canadian Union of Public Employees, 2009) to social policy experts (Zuberi, 2013), to Canadian experts in infection control in hospitals (Zoutman, Ford, & Sopha, 2014) contend that a focus on hand hygiene alone is less effective than a multifaceted approach that considers, for example, hospital cleaning and staffing in attempts to reduce HAI. While many medical experts claim strong evidence for the hand hygiene-HAI link, others are equivocal (e.g. Beggs, Shepherd, & Kerr, 2008; Bryce et al., 2014, p. 710; Jumaa, 2005). The most recent Cochrane review was 'unable to provide clear evidence of the effect of interventions to promote hand hygiene compliance or reduce HAIs' (Gould, Moralejo, Drey, & Chudleigh, 2010, p 10–11). Thus, while no one seems to oppose hand hygiene, its promotion as the solution to HAI is somewhat contested in the medical literature.

But in this sample of newspaper coverage, even articles that discussed other factors in disease transmission still tended to emphasize individual handwashing as the primary solution. Articles that hardly mentioned handwashing in the body of the text often featured handwashing in the headline. A minority of articles pose critical questions about hand hygiene and its promotion. But overall, Canadian newspapers imply that conscientious handwashing alone can stop epidemics and healthcare-associated infection – despite the acknowledged failure of efforts to improve hand hygiene compliance rates long-term, especially when they focus on individual behaviour alone (Wilson et al., 2011). Although the 'just wash your hands' approach seems not be working, alternative approaches tend to be framed as bad science or bad citizenship. This reinforces Wilkins (1993) argument that news media present coverage of scientific issues 'stripped of social, economic and political context' and discuss risks 'in terms of specific people, governments or corporations to "blame," rather than more deeply examining the political and economic system which makes decisions about risk' (p. 74).

Conclusion

News coverage is not a perfect measure of the relevance of health issues. The medical literature on hand hygiene continues to grow, despite the reduction in news coverage. Despite massive efforts in healthcare to reduce HAI through the hiring of experts, the aggressive promotion of hand hygiene and other measures, HAI remains a major concern in Canada. Data on the problem remain incomplete, out of date and unreliable, making it difficult to ascertain what progress has been made (Blackwell, 2015). However, a recent analysis suggests that hospital-associated infection, particularly *C. difficile* and urinary tract infections, increased from 2002 to 2009 in Canada (Taylor et al., 2016). Hand hygiene campaigns do not seem to have solved the HAI problem. Given the movement of HAI from an explicit trigger in the peak years of hand hygiene coverage to a background issue in the waning coverage of later years, it may be that the prominence of the issue of HAI has made articles about hand hygiene itself somewhat obsolete. Further research is necessary to test this hypothesis: did headline news coverage of HAI itself take off as coverage of hand hygiene declined? Does coverage turn toward infection rates in hospitals instead of providers' hand hygiene, and what implications does this have for representations of hand hygiene and infectious diseases? Might more structural analyses rise to the fore?

At least up to 2015, hand hygiene coverage in the news mirrors the general trend toward individual-ization of responsibility in public health (Ayo, 2012; Lindsay, 2010; Raphael, 2008; Thompson & Kumar, 2011). For thirty years, Canadian newspapers have lamented the failure of individuals to wash their hands, while continuing to promote individual hand hygiene as the primary solution to infection. In healthcare facilities, persistent low hand hygiene compliance rates (Luangasanatip et al., 2015) have trig-gered a shift toward holding individual workers accountable for poor hand hygiene (McInnes, Phillips, Middleton, & Gould, 2014, p. 2). The focus on the individual does not seem to be abating.

There are several problems with the message that infectious disease can be curbed or spread by individual hand washers alone. First, it disregards contradictory evidence. Canadian news coverage largely ignores debates within medicine about the evidence base for hand hygiene as a prophylactic against infection. The coverage implies there is universal agreement among experts that handwashing will solve the problem of infection, which is misleading.

Second, individualization may foster resistance. In their analysis of resistance to health promotion campaigns, Thompson and Kumar (2011) note that a focus on irresponsible individuals 'may reinforce the potential for these stigmatized individuals to actively resist the constant health messages telling them how they should act' (p. 114). The medical literature contains plenty of evidence of healthcare providers' resistance to hand hygiene campaigns, documenting message fatigue, exasperation with the campaigns' failure to recognize the structural realities of practice, and the fact that physicians, particu-larly specialists, are less likely to perform or advocate hand hygiene than lower status providers (Jang et al., 2010; McInnes et al., 2014; Pittet et al., 2004; White et al., 2015). Incessantly blaming providers could reduce hand hygiene compliance.

Third, focusing on individual behaviours oversimplifies complex problems in public health. It means we pay inadequate attention to the larger context which constrains and shapes individual behav-iour. Existing power relations and structural constraints make it difficult for patients to ask healthcare providers to wash, and for providers to wash at every possible 'hand hygiene moment' in their busy workday. Focusing on individual hand washers may be cheap and easy, but other factors have been identified which may increase the spread and virulence of infection; these include inadequate funding for healthcare, research and public health; the use of antibacterial products and antibiotics (especially in food animals); issues in hospitals with overcrowding, patient-provider ratios, funding cutbacks and outdated and inadequate facilities (Huttner et al., 2013; Knoll, Lautenschlaeger, & Borneff-Lipp, 2010; McDevitt, 2009; Nosocomial & Occupational Infections Section, 2010; Weber & Hughes, 2004; Zoutman et al., 2014). Targeting individual handwashing deflects attention from such issues, which may implicate health authorities, government agencies and industry, and could lead the public to assess responsibility differently (Kim et al., 2010). If social issues beyond individuals' control affect the spread of infection, it is not only unfair to place responsibility for infection control solely in the hands of individuals; it is an approach that will fail. Less simplistic reporting would help to explain why hand hygiene compliance rates remain low despite considerable effort, why the problems of infectious disease and HAI do not admit of easy solutions, and why other measures to reduce infectious disease may be worthy of public support.

Notes

1. While the World Health Organization uses the abbreviation HCAI, the most common abbreviation for healthcare-associated infection in Canada is HAI (see http://www.phac-aspc.gc.ca/cphorsphc-respcacsp/2013/infections-eng.php).
2. *The Globe & Mail* (published in Toronto) ranked first, *The Toronto Star* second and *The Ottawa Citizen* fifth. The Major Newspapers search function is unavailable in the version of LexisNexis to which the author's university now subscribes. However, in a Major World Publications search conducted in June 2017, *The Globe & Mail* and *The Toronto Star* ranked fifth and sixth, while British papers occupied the top four positions. It appears that hand hygiene peaked in British papers some years after American, Australian and Canadian coverage peaked.

3. Health is primarily under provincial jurisdiction in Canada; while other federalist countries such as the US and Australia have similarly distributed jurisdiction over health, they have more prominent federal public health agencies than Canada (National Advisory Committee on SARS & Public Health, 2003).

Acknowledgments

The author thanks Susan Haydt for assistance in the initial phases of the research, and Howard Ramos, the editors, and two anonymous reviewers for their helpful suggestions.

Disclosure statement

No potential conflict of interest was reported by the author.

Funding

This work was supported by the Nova Scotia Health Research Foundation.

ORCID

Emma Whelan 🆔 http://orcid.org/0000-0002-5276-1907

References

Aunger, R., Schmidt, W.-P., Ranpura, A., Coombes, Y., Maina, P. M., Matiko, C., & Curtis, V. (2010). Three kinds of psychological determinants for hand-washing behaviour in Kenya. *Social Science & Medicine, 70*(3), 383–391.

Ayo, N. (2012). Understanding health promotion in a neoliberal climate and the making of health conscious citizens. *Critical Public Health, 22*(1), 99–105. doi:10.1080/09581596.2010.520692

Barnes, M. D., Hanson, C. L., Novilla, L. M. B., Meacham, A. T., McIntyre, E., & Erickson, B. C. (2008). Analysis of media agenda setting during and after Hurricane Katrina: Implications for emergency preparedness, disaster response, and disaster policy. *American Journal of Public Health, 98*(4), 604–610.

Baron, E. (2011, August 3). 'No excuse' for not washing; Compliance with hygiene rules found lower than 50 per cent in two regions. *The Vancouver Province*, p. A4.

Bashford, A. (2004). *Imperial hygiene: A critical history of colonialism, nationalism and public health*. Basingstoke: Palgrave Macmillan.

Beggs, C. B., Shepherd, S. J., & Kerr, K. G. (2008). Increasing the frequency of hand washing by healthcare workers does not lead to commensurate reductions in staphylococcal infection in a hospital ward. *BMC Infectious Diseases, 8*(1), 641. doi:10.1186/1471-2334-8-114

Bexell, M. (2013). Hand in hand? UN-business cooperation for health and development. *Innovation: The European Journal of Social Science Research, 26*(3), 201–213. doi:10.1080/13511610.2013.771877

Bjerke, N. B. (2004). The evolution: Handwashing to hand hygiene guidance. *Critical Care Nursing Quarterly, 27*(3), 295–307.

Blackwell, T. (2015, January 19). Infected and undocumented: Thousands of Canadians dying from hospital-acquired bugs. *The National Post*. Retrieved from http://news.nationalpost.com/health/infected-and-undocumented-thousands-of-canadians-dying-from-hospital-acquired-bugs?__lsa=2c95-4153

Boyce, J. M., & Pittet, D. (2002). Guideline for hand hygiene in health-care settings: Recommendations of the healthcare infection control practices advisory committee and the HICPAC/SHEA/APIC/IDSA hand hygiene task force. *CDC Morbidity & Mortality Weekly Report, 51*(RR-16), 1–44. Retrieved from https://www.cdc.gov/MMWR/Preview/mmwrhtml/rr5116a1.htm

Braid, D. (2008, January 17). 'No-brainer' hand-washing lesson costs taxpayer $16 M [column]. *The Calgary Herald*, p. A4.

Brown, K. M. (2011). *Foul bodies: Cleanliness in early America*. New Haven, CT: Yale University Press.

Brown, B., Crawford, P., Nerlich, B., & Koteyko, N. (2008). The habitus of hygiene: Discourses of cleanliness and infection control in nursing work. *Social Science & Medicine, 67*(7), 1047–1055.

Brown, B., Nerlich, B., Crawford, P., Koteyko, N., & Carter, R. (2009). Hygiene and biosecurity: The language and politics of risk in an era of emerging infectious diseases. *Sociology Compass, 3*(5), 811–823.

Bryce, E., Islam, S., Nelson, B., Gamage, B., Wilson, R., Welsh, P., & Han, G. (2014). Impact of a mandated provincial hand hygiene program: Messages from the field. *American Journal of Infection Control, 42*(7), 708–712. doi:10.1016/j.ajic.2014.04.004

Burnstein, D. E. (2006). *Next to godliness: Confronting dirt and despair in progressive era New York City*. Urbana, IL: University of Illinois Press.

Butler-Jones, D. (2013). *The chief public health officer's report on the state of public health in Canada, 2013: Infectious disease-the never-ending threat*. Ottawa: Public Health Agency of Canada. Retrieved from https://www.canada.ca/content/dam/phac-aspc/migration/phac-aspc/cphorsphc-respcacsp/2013/assets/pdf/2013-eng.pdf

Campkin, B., & Cox, R. (Eds.). (2013). *Dirt: New geographies of cleanliness and contamination*. London: I. B. Tauris.

Canadian Union of Public Employees. (2009, January). *Healthcare associated infections: A cbackgrounder*. Retrieved from http://cupe.ca/sites/cupe/files/healthcare-associated-infections-cupe-backgrounder.pdf

Conover, J. R., & Laird, J. L. (1921). Hand disinfection – An investigation of various preparations for this purpose. *American Journal of Public Health, 11*(9), 816–824.

Contzen, N., Meili, I. H., & Mosler, H.-J. (2015). Changing handwashing behaviour in southern Ethiopia: A longitudinal study on infrastructural and commitment interventions. *Social Science & Medicine, 124*, 103–114. doi:10.1016/j.socscimed.2014.11.006

Crawford, P., & Brown, B. (2008). Soft authority: Ecologies of infection management in the working lives of modern matrons and infection control staff. *Sociology of Health & Illness, 30*(5), 756–771.

Curtis, V., Biran, A., Deverell, K., Hughes, C., Bellamy, K., & Drasar, B. (2003). Hygiene in the home: Relating bugs and behaviour. *Social Science & Medicine, 57*(4), 657–672.

Dube, R. (2007, June 12). Scalpel? Check. Clean hands? Not so much; Washing up saves lives. So why do doctors and nurses regularly skip the sink between patients? *The Globe and Mail*, p. L1.

Federal/Provincial/Territorial Special Task Force on Public Health. (2005, March). *Partners in public health: Final report*. Ottawa: Health Canada. Retrieved from http://www.phac-aspc.gc.ca/publicat/healthpartners/pdf/partnersinhealthmainreport_e.pdf

Gifford-Jones, D. (1995, December 31). Hand washing – It's the right thing to do [Physician's column]. *The Montreal Gazette*, p. C4.

Gillies, D. (2005). Hempelian and Kuhnian approaches in the philosophy of medicine: The Semmelweis case. *Studies in History and Philosophy of Biological and Biomedical Sciences, 36*, 159–181.

Gould, D. J., Moralejo, D., Drey, N., & Chudleigh, J. H. (2010). Interventions to improve hand hygiene compliance in patient care. *Cochrane Database of Systematic Reviews, 9*, CD005186. doi: 10.1002/14651858.CD005186.pub3

Greenberg, M. R., Sachsman, D. B., Sandman, P. M., & Salomone, K. L. (1989). Network evening news coverage of environmental risk. *Risk Analysis, 9*(1), 119–126. doi:10.1111/j.1539-6924.1989.tb01227.x

Holmes, B. (2009). Media coverage of Canada's obesity epidemic: Illustrating the subtleties of surveillance medicine. *Critical Public Health, 19*(2), 223–233. doi:10.1080/09581590802478048

Hoy, S. (1995). *Chasing dirt: The American pursuit of cleanliness*. New York, NY: Oxford University Press.

Hughes, R. (1995, February 24). Obsession with germs finds justification in Handwashing Week; Pathogenically-correct reporter offers tips on breaking 'cycle of infection.' *The Hamilton Spectator*, p. B3.

Hunt, A. (1999). *Governing morals: A social history of moral regulation*. Cambridge: Cambridge University Press.

Hunt, A. (2003). Risk and moralization in everyday life. In R. V. Ericson & A. Doyle (Eds.), *Risk and morality* (pp. 165–192). Toronto: University of Toronto Press.

Huttner, A., Harbarth, S., Carlet, J., Cosgrove, S., Goossens, H., Holmes, A., ... Pittet, D. (2013). Antimicrobial resistance: A global view from the 2013 World Healthcare-Associated Infections Forum. *Antimicrobial Resistance and Infection Control, 2*(31). Retrieved from http://www.aricjournal.com/content/2/1/31

Ibrahim, M. (2014, November 26). Health staff slip up on handwashing; One-in-four chance your doctor or nurse hasn't, AHS says. *The Edmonton Journal*, p. A3.

Jang, T.-H., Wu, S., Kirzner, D., Moore, C., Youssef, G., Tong, A., ... McGeer, A. (2010). Focus group study of hand hygiene practice among healthcare workers in a teaching hospital in Toronto, Canada. *Infection Control and Hospital Epidemiology, 31*(2), 144–150. doi:10.1086/649792

Juhila, K., Raitakari, S., & Löfstrand, C. H. (2017). Responsibilization in governmentality literature. In K. Juhila, S. Raitakari, & C. Hall (Eds.), *Responsibilisation at the margins of welfare services* (pp. 11–34). London: Routledge.

Jumaa, P. A. (2005). Hand hygiene: Simple and complex. *International Journal of Infectious Diseases, 9*, 3–14. doi:10.1016/j.ijid.2004.05.005

Kelley, V. (2010). *Soap and water: Cleanliness, dirt and the working classes in Victorian and Edwardian Britain*. London: I. B. Tauris.

Kim, A. E., Kumanyika, S., Shive, D., Igweatu, U., & Kim, S. (2010). Coverage and framing of racial and ethnic health disparities in US newspapers, 1996–2005. *American Journal of Public Health, 100*, S224–S231. doi:10.2105/AJPH.2009.171678

Knight Ridder Newspapers. (1998, April 23). School children should learn importance of hand-washing. *The Calgary Herald*, p. W6.

Knoll, M., Lautenschlaeger, C., & Borneff-Lipp, M. (2010). The impact of workload on hygiene compliance in nursing. *British Journal of Nursing, 19*(16), S18–S22. doi:10.12968/bjon.2010.19.Sup6.78213

Koteyko, N., Nerlich, B., Crawford, P., & Wright, N. (2008). 'Not rocket science' or 'No silver bullet'? Media and government discourses about MRSA and cleanliness. *Applied Linguistics, 29*(2), 223–243. doi:10.1093/applin/amn006

Langford, R., & Panter-Brick, C. (2013). A health equity critique of social marketing: Where interventions have impact but insufficient reach. *Social Science & Medicine, 83*, 133–141.

Lindsay, J. (2010). Healthy living guidelines and the disconnect with everyday life. *Critical Public Health, 20*(4), 475–487. doi:10.1080/09581596.2010.505977

London School of Hygiene and Tropical Medicine. (2000). *The global market for soaps: A market research report for the public-private partnership on handwashing with soap*. Retrieved from http://www.bvsde.paho.org/bvsacd/cd27/globalmarketsoap.pdf

Luangasanatip, N., Hongsuwan, M., Limmathurotsakul, D., Lubell, Y., Lee, A. S., Harbarth, S., ... Cooper, B. S. (2015). Comparative efficacy of interventions to promote hand hygiene in hospital: Systematic review and network meta-analysis. *British Medical Journal, 351*, doi:10.1136/bmj.h3728

McCarter, J. (2008, September). *Special report: Prevention and control of hospital-acquired infections*. Toronto: Office of the Auditor General of Ontario. Retrieved from http://www.auditor.on.ca/en/content/specialreports/specialreports/hai_en.pdf

McDevitt, M. (2009, October 8). Editorial: Handwashing. *The Sherbrooke Record*, p. 6.

McInnes, E., Phillips, R., Middleton, S., & Gould, D. (2014). A qualitative study of senior hospital managers' views on current and innovative strategies to improve hand hygiene. *BMC Infectious Diseases, 14*(1), 611. doi:10.1186/s12879-014-0611-3

Miller, P., & Rose, N. (2008). *Governing the present: Administering economic, social and personal life*. Cambridge: Polity Press.

Mowat, D. L., & Butler-Jones, D. (2007). Public health in Canada: A difficult history. *Healthcare Papers, 7*(3), 31–36.

National Advisory Committee on SARS and Public Health. (2003). *Learning from SARS: Renewal of public health in Canada*. Ottawa: Health Canada. Retrieved from http://www.phac-aspc.gc.ca/publicat/sars-sras/pdf/sars-e.pdf

Nerlich, B. (2009). 'The post-antibiotic apocalypse' and the 'war on superbugs': Catastrophe discourse in microbiology, its rhetorical form and political function. *Public Understanding of Science, 18*(5), 574–590. doi:10.1177/0963662507087974

Nicolle, L. (2007). Hygiene: What and why? *Canadian Medical Association Journal, 176*(6), 767–768. doi:10.1503/cmaj.061741

Nosocomial and Occupational Infections Section. (2010). *Essential resources for effective infection prevention and control programs: A matter of patient safety: A discussion paper*. Ottawa: Division of Blood Safety Surveillance and Health Care Acquired Infections, Centre for Communicable Diseases and Infection Control, Public Health Agency of Canada. Retrieved from http://www.phac-aspc.gc.ca/nois-sinp/guide/ps-sp/pdf/ps-sp-eng.pdf

O'Connor, E. (2014, July 9). Hospital hygiene suffers when nobody's watching. *The Vancouver Province*, p. A4.

Ofner, M., Lem, M., Sarwal, S., Vearncombe, M., & Simor, A. (2003). Cluster of severe acute respiratory syndrome cases among protected health-care workers – Toronto, Canada, April 2003. *Morbidity and Mortality Weekly Report, 52*(19), 433–436.

Oliveira, M. (2012, November 19). Keyboards bug-infested; But don't worry, experts say: There's little chance of them making you sick. *The Montreal Gazette*, p. A25.

Ontario Agency for Health Protection and Promotion, & Provincial Infectious Diseases Advisory Committee. (2012). *Best practices for infection prevention and control programs in all health care settings* (3rd ed.). Toronto: Queen's Printer for Ontario. Retrieved from http://www.publichealthontario.ca/fr/eRepository/BP_IPAC_Ontario_HCSettings_2012.pdf.

Ottawa Public Health. (2009, September). Ottawa's health is in your hands. Retrieved from http://documents.ottawa.ca/sites/documents.ottawa.ca/files/documents/con046693.pdf

Parini, S. (2003). Action stat: Severe acute respiratory syndrome. *Nursing, 33*(9), 96.

Pittet, D., Simon, A., Hugonnet, S., Pessoa-Silva, C., Sauvan, V., & Perneger, T. V. (2004). Hand hygiene among physicians: Performance, beliefs, and perceptions. *Annals of Internal Medicine, 141*(1), 1–8. doi:10.7326/0003-4819-141-1-200407060-00008

Plyushteva, A. (2009). This benevolent hand gives you soap: Reflections on global handwashing day from an international development perspective. *Journal of Health Management, 11*(2), 419–430.

Raphael, D. (2008). Grasping at straws: A recent history of health promotion in Canada. *Critical Public Health, 18*(4), 483–495. doi:10.1080/09581590802443604

Raymer, R. (2000, September 21). Letter to the editor: Canada's Upper Hand. *The Globe and Mail*, p. A16.

Silversides, A. (2009). Public reports of infection rates urged. *Canadian Medical Association Journal, 181*(9), 573–574. doi:10.1503/cmaj.109-3056

Smith, V. (2007). *Clean: A history of personal hygiene and purity*. Oxford: Oxford University Press.

Stachenko, S., Legowski, B., & Geneau, R. (2009). Improving Canada's response to public health challenges: The creation of a new public health agency. In R. Beaglehole & R. Bonita (Eds.), *Global public health: A new era* (2nd ed., pp. 123–137). New York, NY: Oxford University Press.

Stow, M. B. K. (Ed.). (2012). *Rome, pollution and propriety: Dirt, disease and hygiene in the eternal city from antiquity to modernity*. Cambridge: Cambridge University Press.

Talaga, T. (2008, October 22). Contract cleaning in hospitals decried; Union leader calls it a 'dangerous practice,' at time when province is working to reduce infection rates. *The Toronto Star*, p. A23.

Taylor, G., Gravel, D., Matlow, A., Embree, J., LeSaux, N., Johnston, L., ... Wong, A. (2016). Assessing the magnitude and trends in hospital acquired infections in Canadian hospitals through sequential point prevalence surveys. *BMC Antimicrobial Resistance & Infection Control, 5*(1), 160. doi:10.1186/s13756-016-0118-3

Thompson, L., & Kumar, A. (2011). Responses to health promotion campaigns: Resistance, denial and othering. *Critical Public Health, 21*(1), 105–117. doi:10.1080/09581591003797129

Vancouver Sun/Canwest News Service. (2009, October 2). Sudsing up may not stem spread of flu; Contentious study dismisses preventive benefit of vigorous handwashing. *The Edmonton Journal*, p. A5.

VanSteelandt, A., Conly, J., Ghali, W., & Mather, C. (2015). Implications of design on infection prevention and control practice in a novel hospital unit: The Medical Ward of the 21st Century. *Anthropology & Medicine, 22*(2), 149–161. doi:10.1080/13648470.2014.1003795

Vigarello, G. (2008). *Concepts of cleanliness: Changing attitudes in France since the Middle Ages.* (J. Birrell Trans.). Cambridge: Cambridge University Press.

Vihos, J. (2014, November 28). Letters: Who is not complying? *The Edmonton Journal,* p. A25

Washer, P., & Joffe, H. (2006). The 'hospital superbug': Social representations of MRSA. *Social Science & Medicine, 63*(8), 2141–2152. doi:10.1016/j.socscimed.2006.05.018

Weber, J. T., & Hughes, J. M. (2004). Beyond Semmelweis: Moving infection control into the community. *Annals of Internal Medicine, 140*(5), 397–398.

White, K. M., Jimmieson, N. L., Obst, P. L., Graves, N., Barnett, A., Cockshaw, W., … Paterson, D. (2015). Using a theory of planned behaviour framework to explore hand hygiene beliefs at the '5 critical moments' among Australian hospital-based nurses. *BMC Health Services Research, 15,* 615. doi:10.1186/s12913-015-0718-2

Wilkins, L. (1993). Between facts and values: Print media coverage of the greenhouse effect, 1987–1990. *Public Understanding of Science, 2*(1), 71–84.

Wilson, S., Jacob, C. J., & Powell, D. (2011). Behavior-change interventions to improve hand-hygiene practice: A review of alternatives to education. *Critical Public Health, 21*(1), 119–127. doi:10.1080/09581591003786122

World Health Organization. (2011). *Report on the Burden of endemic health care-associated infection worldwide: A systematic review of the literature.* Geneva: Author. Retrieved from http://apps.who.int/iris/bitstream/10665/80135/1/9789241501507_eng.pdf

Zhang, Y., Jin, Y., Stewart, S., & Porter, J. (2016). Framing responsibility for depression: How U.S. news media attribute causal and problem-solving responsibilities when covering a major public health problem. *Journal of Applied Communication Research, 44*(2), 118–135. doi:10.1080/00909882.2016.1155728

Zoutman, D. E., Ford, B. D., & Sopha, K. (2014). Environmental cleaning resources and activities in Canadian acute care hospitals. *American Journal of Infection Control, 42*(5), 490–494. doi:10.1016/j.ajic.2014.01.013

Zuberi, D. (2013). *Cleaning up: How hospital outsourcing is hurting workers and endangering patients.* Ithaca, NY: Cornell University Press.

Newspaper, Province of publication	Period archived in Lexis/Nexis	Number of handwashing articles in sample	Number of handwashing articles published before 2000
The Globe & Mail, Ontario	November 1977-present	57	4
The Ottawa Citizen, Ontario	October 1985-present	41	4
The Edmonton Journal, Alberta	April 1989-present	36	0
The Calgary Herald, Alberta	July 1991-present	36	11
The Toronto Star, Ontario	September 1985-present	35	8
The Hamilton Spectator, Ontario	October 1991-present	27	7
The Montreal Gazette, Quebec	April 1985-present	26	7
The Vancouver Sun, British Columbia	July 1991-present	24	1
The Kitchener-Waterloo Record, Ontario	October 1990-present	19	1
The National Post, Ontario	March 1999-present	19	0
The New Brunswick Times & Transcript, New Brunswick	January 1998-present	18	0
The Victoria Times-Colonist, British Columbia	January 2000-present	17	n/a
The Windsor Star, Ontario	January 2000-present	16	n/a
The Nanaimo Daily News, British Columbia	January 2006-present	15	n/a
The Vancouver Province, British Columbia	January 2000-present	14	n/a
TOTALS		400	43

6 Diet, exercise…*and* drugs

Social constructions of healthy lifestyles in weight-related prescription drug advertisements

Crystal Adams and Brittany M. Harder

ABSTRACT

Much research has examined the social constructions of overweightness and obesity in the broader society. This paper aims to contribute to this literature by examining the popular constructions of lifestyle behavior in direct-to-consumer advertising (DTCA) geared toward overweight and obese individuals. We are centrally interested in how pharmaceutical advertisements frame healthy behaviors as a solution to the experience of overweightness and in distinguishing how this framing differs from dominant discourses of health and obesity. We employ ethnographic content analysis to examine the healthy lifestyle discourses of 120 consumer-directed television ads for weight-related conditions. We identify two types of healthy lifestyle ads: (1) drug compliance ads, where behavioral changes around health management are largely restricted to the use of drugs, and (2) complementary drug use ads, where drug use and other types of healthy behaviors, such as diet and exercise, are regarded as essential components to a treatment regimen plan. In all ads, DTCA regards prescription drug adoption as a type of behavior change that, like diet and exercise, is necessary to minimize health risks. We find that to promote drugs, the pharmaceutical industry encourages lifestyle changes, and they do so by simultaneously drawing on and expanding upon the dominant public health discourse around healthy behavior. In finding that pharmaceutical companies frame drug use as a necessary component for overweight and obese individuals' health management, this research contributes to the vast literature that problematizes normative views of the nature, causes, and treatment of obesity and weight-related conditions.

Introduction

Over the past several decades, health professionals, public health practitioners, corporations, and others have declared obesity to be an 'epidemic' in the United States (Campos, Saguy, Ernsberger, Oliver, & Gaesser, 2006; Rich & Evans, 2005; Wright, 2009). The dominant discourses around fat, which claim that fat is a threat to health, have heightened public anxiety around obesity and generated negative attitudes toward overweight and obese individuals. Medicalization reinforces public fear over the threat of fat to health. Notably, the American Medical Association has labeled obesity as a 'disease,' a move that has been highly contested since its introduction in 2013 and which Sadler (2014) contends is 'perhaps the most profound act of medicalization in American medicine' (p. 143). This alarmist rhetoric contrasts with research indicating that excess fat alone is not associated with poorer health; for example, Flegal,

Kit, Orpana, and Graubard (2013) found that overweightness (BMI of 25–<30) was associated with a significantly lower all-cause mortality, and grade 1 (BMI of 30–<35) of obesity was not associated with higher mortality. The medicalization of obesity has relied on social constructions in the media that portrays fatness as a serious problem and one that is best resolved through lifestyle changes. Critical obesity researchers have challenged such constructions in the media.

In the United States, one of the most common forms of health promotion is the direct-to-consumer advertising (DTCA) of prescription drugs. Through DTCA, pharmaceutical companies bring to the public's attention disease and treatment information and the importance of patients' involvement in health decision-making. Up until 1997, consumers received limited information from pharmaceutical companies about their products. Though the FDA did not specifically outlaw the direct-to-consumer marketing of prescription drugs, regulations required such a stringent disclosure of risk information that broadcast advertising was infeasible. This changed in the late 1990s, when the drug industry successfully lobbied the FDA to weaken its risk disclosure requirements in broadcast advertisements. These regulatory changes led to a rapid rise in pharmaceutical marketing activities directed at consumers (Donohue, Cevasco, & Rosenthal, 2007; Palumbo & Mullins, 2002).

Up until now, DTCA research has not examined how DTCA depicts overweightness and obesity, nor has it investigated DTCA's portrayal of acceptable solutions to the supposed problem of fatness. This paper aims to contribute to the critical obesity literature that questions the media's portrayal of overweightness and obesity by investigating the popular constructions of lifestyle behavior in DTCA geared toward overweight and obese individuals. We are centrally interested in how pharmaceutical advertisements frame healthy behaviors as a solution to overweightness and obesity, and in distinguishing how this framing differs from dominant discourses of health and fatness.

The social construction of obesity in the media

Much research investigating the social construction of obesity in the media is grounded in critical obesity scholarship (Boero, 2012; Campos, 2004; Gard & Wright, 2005; Jutel, 2006; Monaghan, 2005; Saguy, 2013; Wright & Harwood, 2009) which critiques the dominant and popular discourses that frame how fat is viewed, treated, and discussed. Many of these scholars have critically analyzed the influence the media has had in constructing the supposed 'obesity epidemic.' For example, Boero (2013) argued that the media does not simply report on already existent social phenomena but rather create new phenomena (p. 371). The media simultaneously reflects and dramatizes traditional biomedical conceptions of the nature, causes, and resolution of obesity as a disease (Saguy & Almeling, 2008).

Previous literature has focused on the media's portrayals of overweightness and obesity, including those in print (Barry, Jarlenski, Grob, Schlesinger, & Gollust, 2011; Boero, 2007; Gollust, Eboh, & Barry, 2012; Kim & Willis, 2007), on television (Barry et al., 2011; Himes & Thompson, 2007; Kim & Willis, 2007; Varava, 2016), and, more recently, online (Bresnahan, Zhuang, Anderson, Zhu, & Viken, 2016; Chou, Prestin, & Kunath, 2014; Heuer, McClure, & Puhl, 2011; Puhl, Peterson, DePierre, & Luedicke, 2013; Yoo & Kim, 2012). Broadly, portrayals of overweight and obese persons in the media are largely negative and are imbued with unfavorable judgments about their character (Petersen & Lupton, 1996). Overweight persons are portrayed as lacking the will, knowledge, and motivation required to manage weight (LeBesco, 2011; Saguy & Gruys, 2010; Smith & Holm, 2010). Biomedical standards underlie notions of healthy behaviors, and a lack of compliance with these standards is considered moral failure. Though overweightness and obesity is common in the United States, these portrayals have contributed to the stigmatization of overweight and obese persons.

Critical obesity scholars have also problematized normative views of weight-loss treatments. As Jutel (2006) has noted, obesity's categorization as a disease is accompanied by targeted actions aimed at addressing overweightness and obesity with the goal of eliminating it. Dominant obesity discourse focuses on individual-level behaviors as the cause and, thus, the resolution of the obesity epidemic (Atanasova, Koteyko, & Gunter, 2012; Chaufan, Yeh, Ross, & Fox, 2015; Shugart, 2013). Through this perspective, causal 'energy-in, energy-out' explanations of weight are reinforced as the dominant perspective. Overweight and obese individuals are often scrutinized and are pressured to engage in lifestyle and behavior modifications such as diet and exercise. This framing allows profit-seeking industries to market products that claim to encourage healthy choices and health-promoting behaviors.

Healthy lifestyles and DTCA

To the authors' knowledge, only one study has examined the healthy lifestyle content of DTCA. Byrne, Niederdeppe, Avery, and Cantor (2013) found that DTCA provides mixed messages about the efficacy of diet and exercise in reducing the risk of high cholesterol and heart disease, simultaneously depicting individuals relying in vain on diet and exercise to control their cholesterol levels yet also emphasizing the importance of diet and exercise (Byrne et al., 2013). Most research that has examined healthy lifestyles and DTCA has focused on the effects of exposure to DTCA on consumer intentions to adopt a healthy lifestyle. Mathur, Gould, and Khazeni (2016) found an interesting yet unexpected relationship between exposure to DTCA and consumer intentions: advertisement exposure led to higher intentions to apply lifestyle changes relative to drug adoption. This research opposes findings from an earlier study (Bolton, Reed, Volpp, & Armstrong, 2008), which reported that DTCA reduces intentions to engage in healthy behaviors. Recently, Kruger, Niederdeppe, Byrne, and Avery (2015) reported that DTCA for drugs aimed to reduce high cholesterol and heart disease evoked consumer feelings of guilt regarding food and exercise. Although previous research gives some insight into DTCA messages of diet and exercise, their analysis is limited to cholesterol management drugs. Further, their sample of ads is somewhat outdated, with the inclusion of print ads between 1994 and 2005 and television ads between 1999 and 2007 in Byrne et al.'s study, and ads from 2000 to 2007 in Kruger et al.'s (2015) study.

Methods

Considering our primary interest in the healthy lifestyle portrayals in DTCA aimed at overweight and obese persons, we analyze the lifestyle discourses of 120 consumer-directed television advertisements for weight-related conditions. Because DTCA on television is currently one of the most pervasive forms of health promotion, it is important to examine their healthy lifestyle messages, particularly for weight-related DTCA. While we understand that the categories 'overweight' and 'obese' are clinically distinct, it is not clear whether these two diagnoses are experienced differently. Nor is it clear whether advertisers make clinical distinctions when designing advertisements. Thus, our coding process does not distinguish between 'overweight' and 'obese' unless these terms are explicitly used in the advertisement. This is in line with our critical obesity approach, which questions the clinical boundaries around excessive weight.

Data

Advertisements were accessed through AdPharm, an online database of healthcare and pharmaceutical communications. The data included in this study are prescription drug advertisements aimed to treat weight-related conditions that aired on television in the United States from 1997 to 2015. We identified weight-related conditions using the National Institutes of Health's (NIH) list of weight-related conditions (National Institutes of Health [NIH], 2016). This list includes advertisements for drugs aimed to treat heart disease, high blood pressure, stroke, type II diabetes, metabolic syndrome, cancer, osteoarthritis, sleep apnea, gallstones, and reproductive problems. Although other conditions not listed here may be considered weight-related, the NIH's list provides weight-related conditions that are widely recognized and agreed upon. We also included advertisements for cholesterol-lowering drugs, since high cholesterol is widely regarded as a risk factor for heart disease, as well as advertisements for pharmaceutical drugs aimed to treat overweightness and obesity.

Table 1. Frequency of promoted conditions and brand name drugs in sample.

Promoted condition	Frequency	Brand name (n)
Acid reflux	12	Nexium (12)
Arthritis	38	Celebrex (9); Vioxx (1); Xeljanz (6); Enbrel (6); Cymbalta (3); Humira (11) Orencia (2)
Atrial fibrillation	14	Eliquis (4); Xarelto (7); Pradaxa (3)
Diabetes	16	Onglyza (1); Levemir (4); NovoLog Flexpen (4); Novo Nordisk (3) Victoza (4)
High cholesterol	34	Crestor (16); Lipitor (15); Vytorin (1); Caduet (2)
High triglycerides	1	Lovaza (1)
Osteoporosis	3	Reclast (3)
Overweightness	1	Belviq (1)
Stroke	1	Pradaxa (1)
Total	120	24

Search strategy

We used AdPharm's advanced search feature, which allowed us to search for DTCA for each weight-related condition. We searched 'DTC USA TV' and keywords for weight-related conditions, such as 'DTC USA TV heart disease' and 'DTCA USA TV high blood pressure.' These searches often yielded advertisements that did not meet our eligibility criteria; therefore, following each search, we scrutinized the advertisements to exclude those that were ineligible. We then excluded any duplicate advertisements that were in our sample. The final sample includes 120 advertisements (see Table 1).

Analysis

The analysis of advertisements was highly iterative, particularly in the first round of coding. This round consisted of the two authors coding 32 advertisements (about ¼ of the final sample) using a coding scheme that was based on Altheide and Schneider's (2012) suggestions for ECA research protocols. Following the first round of coding, we discussed and revised the coding scheme. While some elements of the final coding scheme are quantitative in scope, most other elements are qualitative or thematic. The quantitative elements include the filename of the advertisement, the brand name of the drug, the condition targeted by the treatment, the date aired, the date the ad was added to the AdPharm database, and the ad length. The qualitative elements include the framing of the problem as presented in the ad, a general description of the discourses used to describe the problem (including any standout quotes that were repeated in the advertisement), a description of the images and animation used in the advertisement (including the presence of overweight and/or obese actors and the sociodemographic characteristics of the actors), depictions of the doctor–patient relationship, and an overall summary of the ad. In all the qualitative codes, we devoted attention to the advertisements portrayal' of the relative roles of healthy behaviors versus the drug in effectively managing the condition.

After the final coding scheme was solidified, we divided the remaining 88 advertisements between the two authors to independently code. We met throughout this second stage of coding to discuss our progress and clarify any questions or concerns. We then took a random sample of ten advertisements and each author coded five during the second stage; these advertisements were coded to test for intercoder agreement. Unlike intercoder agreement in more quantitative analyses, our approach follows that of Armstrong, Gosling, Weinman, & Marteau (1997), where the codes are discussed and where each coder's interpretations of the data are challenged. Intercoder agreement enhances the quality of the research to ensure that the analysis reflects more of a shared interpretation of the data rather than an individual one (Armstrong et al. 1997). We found much agreement in our coding, with any differences being due to emphasis rather than genuine disagreement.

Table 2. Frequency of advertisements by type in sample.

Advertisement type	Frequency	Frequency of advertisement with overweight or obese actors	Promoted conditions (n)
Drug compliance	64	6	Acid reflux (12), Arthritis (9), Atrial fibrillation (15), Diabetes (11), High cholesterol (17)
Complementary drug use	56	20	Arthritis (29), Diabetes (5), High cholesterol (17), High triglycerides (1), Osteoporosis (3), Overweightness (1),
Total	120	26	9

Findings

In this section, we describe the healthy lifestyle discourses and their relationship to weight in DTCA. The results reveal two important dimensions of problem resolution as they are presented in DTCA: the role of the drug, and the role of healthy behaviors not involving drug use. We find two forms of healthy lifestyle DTCA advertisements that speak to these two dimensions: (1) drug compliance ads, where behavioral changes pertaining to health management are largely restricted to the use of drugs and (2) complementary drug use ads, where drug use and other types of healthy behaviors, such as diet and exercise, are regarded as essential components to a treatment regimen plan. Regardless of the healthy lifestyle type promoted, advertisements focus on drugs as enabling the user to live a healthy lifestyle. Table 2 details the frequency of advertisements by type in our sample, including the frequency of advertisements with overweight actors and the conditions promoted by advertisement type.

All you need is drugs: drug compliance as action

One type of healthy lifestyle advertisement portrays drug use as the sole component of a healthy lifestyle. In the dominant public health discourse, behavior, and lifestyle in relation to health management are focused on exercise and diet. These 'drug compliance' advertisements, however, attempt to present drug compliance as a *type* of behavioral lifestyle change. The drug is portrayed as the sole solution to the condition, and the type of behavioral changes necessary to improve one's health status are limited to taking the drug. This framing makes condition management equivalent to drug management.

Advertisements usually portray featured patients doing the conventionally correct things to manage their condition but who nonetheless have health problems. These ads very rarely feature individuals already living unhealthy lifestyles. They are usually fit and living an active life. For example, in a Lipitor advertisement, a man is shown racing on a bike in the mountains, while a sign with high cholesterol numbers chases him. In other words, his attempts to manage his cholesterol through exercise are in vain. Another Lipitor advertisement profiles a female basketball player who is happily participating in a basketball game while surrounded by cheering fans. Various 'stats' related to her coaching experience and general good health are disclosed. In other scenes, she is shown being active and eating healthily. Then, another statistic is displayed: 'Total Cholesterol: 277.' A caption states, 'High cholesterol is a tougher opponent than you think…for millions of adults with high cholesterol, diet and exercise aren't always enough.' The message in these Lipitor advertisements is twofold. First, a healthy lifestyle cannot stave off all diseases. Second, external indicators of health, such as weight, are faulty. Thus, thin, fit people who think they are healthy should question their health status and visit their physician to determine their cholesterol levels.

In terms of disease etiology, these advertisements focus on the non-preventable origins of the condition and on how the efforts on the part of the patients to manage the condition without the use of drugs are partially to wholly ineffective. Frequently, advertisements explicitly or implicitly convey the message that genetic factors are the underlying cause of the focal health problem. This enables drug compliance advertisements to either ignore or downplay the role of healthy behaviors not involving drug use, such as diet and exercise, in prevention or disease management. While many drug compliance advertisements include brief statements (in written format or verbally) that explain that the drug should be used alongside diet and exercise, the primary message is that drug use is sufficient to manage health. The advertisements that directly discuss diet and exercise focus on their limitations and often argue that, for many people, behavioral changes have a limited impact. The natural conclusion is that, for these people, drugs are the only way to manage a condition. For example, Pfizer had a 'Stop Kidding' campaign for Lipitor that lasted several years. One advertisement in this campaign featured a fit middle-aged man exercising in a gym. In bold text and voiceovers, the advertisement states, 'Stop Kidding Yourself.' The actor in the advertisement tells the audience, 'Diet and exercise weren't enough for me. I stopped kidding myself. I've been eating healthier, exercising more, and now I'm also taking Lipitor.'

The importance of patient involvement in illness management is not as prominent of a theme in these advertisements, compared to those that devote greater attention to the importance of behavioral changes in resolving health problems. Why? Because the drug has 'got it covered.' In an effort to make drug use attractive, many advertisements emphasize its ease and convenience. In an advertisement for FlexPen, a pre-filled insulin pen designed to ensure insulin injection is convenient and painless, a patient of average weight discusses her diagnosis experience. The day her doctor told her she had diabetes, she realized there was a lot she had to do to manage her illness. Once she discovered FlexPen, she realized there was something she 'didn't have to do anymore.' The advertisement ends with the patient saying that FlexPen is 'insulin delivery, my way.' Additionally, in an advertisement for the anticoagulant Xarelto, the featured patient, an in-shape middle-aged man who is shown participating in various outdoor activities, explains that monthly visits to the clinic are no longer necessary because of Xarelto, which is taken once daily. This allows the profiled patient to be 'on the move.' In these advertisements, health empowerment results from taking the drug rather than from making behavioral changes involving non-drug use.

Complementary drug use: drugs are the primary, but not sole, solution to the condition

Since the pharmaceutical industry profits from the adoption of pharmaceuticals, and behavioral changes might obviate the need for drugs, one might expect DTCA to deny that behavioral changes are significant contributors to chronic illness. As we have seen with the drug compliance advertisements, this is most certainly the case. However, another type of lifestyle advertisement, what we refer to as 'complementary drug use' advertisements, portrays behavioral changes such as diet and exercise in a positive light and as equally important as drug use. These types of behavioral changes are not sufficient to combat health problems, but they are necessary adjuncts to pharmaceuticals. In other words, for many conditions, a completely healthy lifestyle includes diet, exercise, *and* pharmaceuticals. In contrast to the patients in drug compliance ads, these ads are more likely to feature overweight persons.

A Vytorin advertisement, for example, displays a series of images of unhealthy foods, such as pizza and hamburgers, alongside various family members. This advertisement begins with a voiceover that states, 'Vytorin treats two sources: food and family. Eat right, stay active. But if that's not enough, ask your doctor about adding Vytorin.' All of the patients featured in the ad appear to be overweight. A Nexium advertisement goes as far as to provide consumers with a 'purple plus program,' where users can learn about proper nutrition and exercise. The message here is that pharmaceutical use, knowledge, and a healthy lifestyle go hand in hand. Unlike 'drug compliance' advertisements, which focus on the limitations of diet and exercise, complementary drug use advertisements frame diet and exercise in a positive light, thus encouraging the audience to adopt these behavioral changes alongside the advertised product. The message is clear: for many, a completely healthy lifestyle includes drug use.

An ad for the weight loss drug Belviq features overweight men and women during mealtime who are having difficulty deciding whether and how much to eat. The actors' fictional testimonies detail the difficulties involved with solely using willpower to prevent excessive eating. The narrator concludes with the statement, 'Weight loss is not just about willpower. While we have different triggers, we face similar challenges. Maybe it's time to try Belviq.' While the advertisement argues that lifestyle changes alone could not help these patients lose weight, healthy behaviors along with drug use are presented as necessary for good health.

In terms of etiology, complementary drug use advertisements offer a more complex, nuanced view of the causes of disease. The focus is on both the controllable as well as uncontrollable origins of the condition, and unhealthy habits are a key source of health problems. In doing so, these advertisements send a message that is consistent with the dominant public health rhetoric. However, while patients should eat healthily and be physically active, to fully safeguard their health they should talk to their doctor about prescription drug alternatives. To not talk to one's doctor about pharmaceuticals is to take a risk, as other lifestyle changes may not be sufficient to combat health problems. A Lovaza (a drug that reduces triglyceride levels) advertisement describes high triglycerides as being a 'serious medical condition.' The advertisement begins with a statement from a middle-aged White man in a white laboratory coat: 'Lovaza. Where nature meets science.' By invoking the legitimacy of science, and by emphasizing that Lovaza should be taken within the context of a healthy lifestyle, this advertisement seems less like an industry advertisement and more like public health promotion.

As with 'drug compliance' advertisements, some complementary drug use advertisements portray people who appear to be healthy (i.e. thin and in-shape) but still have health problems. However, in these advertisements, the message is that drugs cannot replace a healthy lifestyle and are only one component of good health maintenance. Unlike in drug compliance advertisements, good health is not an automatic effect of drug use, making it essential for patients to adopt a variety of healthy behaviors to be healthy.

Drugs use facilitates healthy lifestyles

While all advertisements can be distinguished into one of the two categories discussed previously, based on the role of diet and exercise in preventing and treating illness, both drug compliance and complementary drug use advertisements have one feature in common: they present drugs as *enabling* patients to adopt healthy behaviors. In other words, a healthy lifestyle is an *effect* of taking a drug, regardless of the role of behavioral changes in causing the onset of a condition. A Celebrex advertisement, for example, features a thin male patient in a picture book, sitting motionless on a bench. The photos in the picture book are initially static, and arthritis is depicted as disabling. When each illustrated page is flipped, showing the man engaged in outdoor activities, it quickly becomes apparent that the man is no longer in pain, presumably because he is taking Celebrex. Though advertisements such as these depict physical activity as an important aspect of a healthy life, they do not attribute a lack of physical activity as the cause of the focal health condition. Instead, the drug enables patients to live a happy, healthy life.

Advertisements vary in their clarity as to how, exactly, drugs can enable patients to maintain a healthy lifestyle. Some drugs, such as those for arthritis, may help individuals adopt behavioral changes. Celebrex, for example, is for osteoarthritis, a disabling disease that makes being physically active difficult. Therefore, by managing the pain and stiffness that comes with arthritis, patients can exercise. The above-mentioned Belviq ad presents the drug as enabling the featured patients to make wise dietary decisions. For other drugs, it is less clear how the product helps patients adopt healthy behaviors, and in their attempt to portray the drug as contributing to a healthy lifestyle, many advertisements associate the drug with false indications. For example, a Victoza (indicated for Type II diabetes) advertisement claims that 'Victoza is not for weight loss but it may help you lose some weight.' Moreover, as stated in a Lipitor advertisement, 'I've been eating healthier, exercising more, and now I'm also taking Lipitor.' Neither Victoza nor Lipitor is indicated for weight loss or for the adoption of healthy behaviors, and the advertisements do not explain how the promoted drug would help patients attain these goals.

Discussion

This study finds that healthy lifestyles are a central component of pharmaceutical advertisements for weight-related conditions. By analyzing the nature of the discourses of healthy lifestyles in DTCA, this study finds that both drug compliance and complementary drug use healthy lifestyle advertisements regard drug use as a type of healthy behavior. The two types of advertisements differ in that drug compliance advertisements either ignore or highlight the inefficacy of non-drug use healthy behaviors such as diet and exercise, whereas complementary drug use advertisements regard both drug use and other types of healthy behaviors as essential components of disease management. In addition, overweight and obese actors are more likely to be featured in complementary drug use advertisements but are relatively absent in drug compliance advertisements. All advertisements go beyond a narrow focus on healthy lifestyles to discuss the positive effects of drug use on patients' lives. The two types of healthy lifestyle advertisements noted here may explain Byrne et al.'s (2013) finding that DTCA contains mixed messages regarding the importance of diet and exercise.

Except for the Belviq ad, weight is not explicitly discussed in the ads. Instead, the importance of keeping a low weight is implied in the discussion of healthy behaviors. The way these individuals are represented is quite different from their portrayal in other media, which unambiguously regard overweightness and obesity as a failure of moral character. In DTCA, the health problems of the overweight and obese are presented as being outside of their control, and they are depicted as trying, though unsuccessfully, to be healthy. Research (Ashmore, Friedman, Reichmann, & Musante, 2008; Puhl & Brownell, 2006; Vartanian & Shaprow, 2008) has shown that negative weight portrayals do not effectively motivate overweight and obese persons to engage in healthy behaviors. The more positive depictions of overweight and obese persons in DTCA may lead this community to feel less stigmatized by conveying the message that even people who try to live healthfully can be unhealthy. However, DTCA's treatment of lifestyle behavior for overweight and obese patients may constitute a new public health moralism around weight that suggests that any solutions to the negative health effects of fatness must be associated with exercise or diet, regardless of how ineffective that strategy may be. This type of moralism may be less stigmatizing but nonetheless invoke subtle notions of individual responsibility and blame.

By presenting drug use as a type of behavioral solution, DTCA draws on the dominant public health discourse concerning the importance of adopting and maintaining healthy behaviors. By defining drug use as a healthy behavior, DTCA appears less like profiteering through corporate-based interests and more like a legitimate, non-biased source of health information. In other words, it somewhat resembles public health promotion, the goal of which is to prevent and manage disease. Many advertisements focus on managing disease rather than emphasizing to patients that they can prevent the onset of a disease or cure an existing disease. For drugs promoted for risk factors for disease, like high cholesterol and high blood pressure, patients are potentially always at risk and control is oriented toward prevention rather than disease management. Our findings support Dumit's (2012) conclusion that the pharmaceutical industry promotes the perception that all patients, even those who are seemingly healthy, are inherently at risk and in need of chronic treatment to minimize this risk. As Geoffrey Rose (1981) has noted, the risk of disease lies on a continuum, and medical diagnoses such as 'hypertension,' 'hypercholesterolemia,' or 'impaired' glucose tolerance are arbitrary distinctions. This arbitrariness opens the door for drug companies to structure their advertisements to make patients believe they are at high-risk for disease.

Embedded in this discourse are notions of what is and is not controllable in terms of the causes of disease. Advertisements present drug use as a healthy behavior that addresses uncontrollable causes of disease, such as genetics, whereas most other healthy behaviors promoted by the dominant public health discourse are preventative in nature. By presenting drug use as a choice within patients' control, a healthy behavior presentation of drug use serves the dual function of making pharmaceuticals seem like controllable causes of disease such as diet and exercise. The controllable aspect is reflected in the choice to take a drug.

DTCA also differs from standard public health promotion. It goes beyond a simple focus on healthy behavior by emphasizing the limitations of healthy behavior. This is necessary for DTCA to sell drugs; if DTCA reduced itself entirely to the logic of public health, it would essentially be promoting prevention, since, after all, the aim of public health is prevention. The pharmaceutical industry cannot maintain a primary focus on prevention, as this negates the need for drugs and, therefore, for a pharmaceutical industry. Further, as previously mentioned, DTCA differs from public health discourse by depicting overweight and obese individuals in a less stigmatizing light.

The representation of the role of healthy lifestyles in disease prevention in both types of advertisements is paradoxical. On the one hand, these advertisements emphasize that healthy lifestyles cannot stave off disease for everyone. Audiences are encouraged to think that they are a part of a select group for which lifestyle changes alone will not thwart disease. On the other hand, the very mention of healthy lifestyles provides legitimacy to the dominant public health paradigm around healthy lifestyles. When drug compliance advertisements contend that diet and exercise may not work for everyone, they unintentionally deliver the message that lifestyle modifications are the best recourse for improving health, and drugs should be considered only when changes in diet and exercise fail. By promoting drugs alongside healthy lifestyles, complementary drug use advertisements underscore the importance of diet and exercise.

DTCA also differs in terms of its definition of health. While public health has been criticized for focusing on individual-level solutions for addressing public health problems (Becker, 1993; Petersen & Lupton, 1996), DTCA reflects a multidimensional view of health similar to well-respected health agencies such as the National Institutes of Health and the World Health Organization. Both agencies define *health* as being 'a state of complete physical, mental and social well-being and not merely the absence of disease or infirmity' (NIH, 2016; World Health Organization [WHO], 2017). Advertisements do not take a narrow view of health that is merely focused on the physical state. Instead, they frame health as encompassing the physical, mental, and social dimensions of well-being. This social aspect is an important dimension of health. Friends and family are shown in advertisements supporting sufferers in the diagnosis and the management of disease, and they are also shown in scenes related to the effects of drug use and illness management on patients' social lives.

Conclusions: limitations and future research

The current study goes beyond the existing literature on the social construction of overweight and obesity and DTCA by analyzing the lifestyle discourses of prescription drug advertisements for weight-related conditions. Interestingly, we did not find variation by advertising strategy in the racial or gender portrayals of the actors. One might have expected, for example, for complementary drug use ads to have had a higher representation of African-Americans or Hispanics compared to drug compliance ads since these minorities experience higher rates of overweightness and obesity. Complementary drug use ads might have had more females given that females experience greater social pressures around weight. This lack of variation is likely due to the perception that excessive weight is a health problem all sociodemographic groups, including Whites and males. Because weight problems are seen as being universal, advertisers likely do not target a specific racial or gender subgroup so as to appeal to as broad of an audience as possible. This finding may not hold for other types of conditions, and researchers should investigate how weight portrayals differ by race and gender in ads for other types of conditions.

Our research has several limitations. First, the advertisements in our sample (except for the Belviq ad) are not solely targeted to the overweight and obese population. There are multiple causes for the conditions in our sample, and being overweight and obese is only one such cause that pharmaceutical companies consider when they design advertisements. In addition, our findings cannot be generalized to advertisements for non-weight-related conditions. Other types of consumer-directed advertisements could be pursued, such as radio and print advertisements, as well as advertisements for other types of weight-related treatments, such as over-the-counter supplements.

Disclosure statement

The authors report no conflicts of interest.

References

Altheide, D. L., & Schneider, C. J. (2012). *Qualitative media analysis* (Vol. 38). Washington, DC: Sage.

Armstrong, D., Gosling, A., Weinman, J., & Marteau, T. (1997). The place of inter-rater reliability in qualitative research: an empirical study. *Sociology, 31*(3), 597–606.

Ashmore, J. A., Friedman, K. E., Reichmann, S. K., & Musante, G. J. (2008). Weight-based stigmatization, psychological distress, & binge eating behavior among obese treatment-seeking adults. *Eating Behaviors, 9*, 203–209.

Atanasova, D., Koteyko, N., & Gunter, B. (2012). Obesity in the news: Directions for future research. *Obesity Reviews, 13*, 554–559.

Barry, C. L., Jarlenski, M., Grob, R., Schlesinger, M., & Gollust, S. E. (2011). News media framing of childhood obesity in the United States from 2000 to 2009. *Pediatrics, Peds*, 2010–3924.

Becker, M. H. (1993). A medical sociologist looks at health promotion. *Journal of Health and Social Behavior, 34*, 1–6.

Boero, N. (2007). All the news that's fat to print: The American Obesity Epidemic" and the media. *Qualitative Sociology, 30*, 41–60.

Boero, N. (2012). *Killer fat: Media, medicine, and morals in the American "Obesity Epidemic"*. New Brunswick, NJ: Rutgers University Press.

Boero, N. (2013). Obesity in the media: Social science weighs in. *Critical Public Health, 23*, 371–380.

Bolton, L. E., Reed, A., Volpp, K. G., & Armstrong, K. (2008). How does drug and supplement marketing affect a healthy lifestyle? *Journal of Consumer Research, 34*, 713–726.

Bresnahan, M., Zhuang, J., Anderson, J., Zhu, Y., & Viken, G. (2016). "Governor of the House of Pancake": A content analysis of the political framing of Chris Christie's size in online news media. *Fat Studies*, 1–15.

Byrne, S., Niederdeppe, J., Avery, R. J., & Cantor, J. (2013). "When diet and exercise are not enough": An examination of lifestyle change inefficacy claims in direct-to-consumer advertising. *Health Communication, 28*, 800–813.

Campos, P. F. (2004). *The obesity myth: Why America's obsession with weight is hazardous to your health*. New York, NY: Penguin.

Campos, P., Saguy, A., Ernsberger, P., Oliver, E., & Gaesser, G. (2006). The epidemiology of overweight and obesity: Public health crisis or moral panic? *International Journal of Epidemiology, 35*, 55–60.

Chaufan, C., Yeh, J., Ross, L., & Fox, P. (2015). You can't walk or bike yourself out of the health effects of poverty: Active school transport, child obesity, and blind spots in the public health literature. *Critical Public Health, 25*, 32–47.

Chou, W.-Y. S., Prestin, A., & Kunath, S. (2014). Obesity in social media: A mixed methods analysis. *Translational Behavioral Medicine, 4*, 314–323.

Donohue, J. M., Cevasco, M., & Rosenthal, M. B. (2007). A decade of direct-to-consumer advertising of prescription drugs. *New England Journal of Medicine, 2007*, 673–681.

Dumit, J. (2012). *Drugs for life: How pharmaceutical companies define our health*. Durham, NC: Duke University Press.

Flegal, K. M., Kit, B. K., Orpana, H., & Graubard, B. I. (2013). Association of all-cause mortality with overweight and obesity using standard body mass index categories: A systematic review and meta-analysis. *Journal of the American Medical Association, 309*, 71–82.

Gard, M., & Wright, J. (2005). *The obesity epidemic: Science, morality and ideology*. New York, NY: Routledge.

Gollust, S. E., Eboh, I., & Barry, C.L. (2012). Picturing obesity: Analyzing the social epidemiology of obesity conveyed through US news media images. *Social Science & Medicine, 74*, 1544–1551.

Heuer, C. A., McClure, K. J., & Puhl, R. M. (2011). Obesity stigma in online news: A visual content analysis. *Journal of Health Communication, 16*, 976–987.

Himes, S. M., & Thompson, J. K. (2007). fat stigmatization in television shows and movies: A content analysis. *Obesity, 15*, 712–718.

Jutel, A. (2006). The emergence of overweight as a disease entity: Measuring up normality. *Social Science & Medicine, 63*, 2268–2276.

Kim, S.-H., & Willis, L. A. (2007). Talking about obesity: News framing of who is responsible for causing and fixing the problem. *Journal of Health Communication, 12*, 359–376.

Kruger, C., Niederdeppe, J., Byrne, S., & Avery, R.J. (2015). Effects of exposure to direct-to-consumer television advertising for statin drugs on food and exercise guilt. *Patient Education and Counseling, 98*, 1150–1155.

LeBesco, K. (2011). Neoliberalism, public health, and the moral perils of fatness. *Critical Public Health, 21*, 153–164.

Mathur, M. B., Gould, M., & Khazeni, N. (2016). Direct-to-consumer drug advertisements can paradoxically increase intentions to adopt lifestyle changes. *Frontiers in Psychology, 7*, 1–11.

Monaghan, L. F. (2005). Discussion piece: A critical take on the obesity debate. *Social Theory & Health, 3*, 302–314.

National Institutes of Health. (2016). What are the health risks of overweight and obesity? Retrieved from https://www.nhlbi.nih.gov/health/health-topics/topics/obe/risks

Palumbo, F. B., & Mullins, C. D. (2002). The development of direct-to-consumer prescription drug advertising regulation. *Food & Drug LJ, 57*, 423–443.

Petersen, A., & Lupton, D. (1996). *The new public health: Health and self in the age of risk*. Thousand Oaks, CA: Sage Publications.

Puhl, R. M., & Brownell, K. D. (2006). Confronting and coping with weight stigma: An investigation of overweight and obese adults. *Obesity, 14*, 1802–1815.

Puhl, R. M., Peterson, J. L., DePierre, J. A., & Luedicke, J. (2013). Headless, hungry, and unhealthy: A video content analysis of obese persons portrayed in online news. *Journal of Health Communication, 18,* 686–702.

Rich, E., & Evans, J. (2005). 'Fat ethics' – The obesity discourse and body politics. *Social Theory & Health, 3,* 341–358.

Rose, G. (1981). Strategy of prevention: Lessons from cardiovascular disease. *British medical journal (Clinical research ed.), 282,* 1847–1851.

Sadler, J. Z. (2014). Risk factor medicalization, hubris, and the obesity disease. *Narrative Inquiry in Bioethics, 4,* 143–146.

Saguy, A. (2013, June). If obesity is a disease, why are so many obese people healthy? *Time,* p. 24.

Saguy, A. C., & Almeling, R. (2008). *Fat in the fire? Science, the news media, and the "Obesity Epidemic" 2.* Paper presented at the Sociological Forum.

Saguy, A. C., & Gruys, K. (2010). Morality and health: News media constructions of overweight and eating disorders. *Social Problems, 57,* 231–250.

Shugart, H. A. (2013). Weight of tradition: Culture as a rationale for obesity in contemporary US news coverage. *Obesity Reviews, 14,* 736–744.

Smith, L. H., & Holm, L. (2010). Social class and body management. A qualitative exploration of differences in perceptions and practices related to health and personal body weight. *Appetite, 55,* 311–318.

Varava, K. (2016). Visual framing, stigmatization, race, and obesity: Examining television news presentation of stories about obesity and stories about health. *Communication Studies, 67,* 509–529.

Vartanian, L. R., & Shaprow, J. G. (2008). Effects of weight stigma on exercise motivation and behavior: A preliminary investigation among college-aged females. *Journal of Health Psychology, 13,* 131–138.

World Health Organization (WHO). (2017) Frequently asked questions. Retrieved from http://www.who.int/suggestions/faq/en/

Wright, J. (2009). Biopower, biopedagogies and the obesity epidemic. In J. Wright & V. Harwood (Eds.), *Biopolitics and the 'obesity epidemic': Governing bodies* (1–14). New York, NY: Routledge.

Wright, J., & Harwood, V. (Eds.). (2009). *Biopolitics and the 'obesity epidemic': Governing bodies* (Vol. 3). New York, NY: Routledge.

Yoo, J. H., & Kim, J. (2012). Obesity in the new media: A content analysis of obesity videos on YouTube. *Health Communication, 27,* 86–97.

7 'I cannot explain it. I knew it was wrong'

A public account of cigarette smoking in pregnancy

Katherine Hodgetts and Shona Helen Crabb

ABSTRACT

In this paper, we examine a situated example of the media's (re)production of shared understandings around smoking, pregnancy and health. Through a discursive lens, we address the way in which Australian media personality Chrissie Swan accounted, on radio, for her continued smoking while pregnant after photographic evidence of her tobacco use entered the public domain. We argue that Swan's account of her smoking privileges a version of 'the good mother' as solely responsible for the health of her foetus, and right to feel ashamed when putting this at risk. A construction of smoking as a (medicalised, irrational) addiction enables her to manage a positive identity in the face of this construction: she presents as being 'thwarted' in her quitting efforts by a force beyond her control. Ultimately, we argue that the version of 'good motherhood' constructed in Swan's account is paradoxical, and may serve both to support, and constrain, pregnant smokers' capacity to sustain quitting behaviours over the long term. In turn, we argue that 'moralising' anti-smoking interventions aimed at pregnant women may be less useful than an approach that interrogates the range of socio-cultural expectations of 'good motherhood' by which pregnant women are simultaneously positioned.

Pregnancy, smoking and 'good motherhood'

In 2013, while pregnant with her third child, Australian media personality Chrissie Swan was followed by a paparazzo who photographed her smoking in her car. After trying (unsuccessfully) to buy the photographs, Swan elected to talk about the incident on radio prior to their publication in a national women's magazine. This radio 'confession' was subsequently discussed and reported in a range of other Australian media contexts, providing a situated example of the media's construction and reproduction of shared understandings around the issues of smoking, pregnancy and motherhood.

Although characterised by an overtly anti-smoking climate, tobacco use remains relatively prevalent in Australia (Weiland, Jelinek, Taylor, & Taylor, 2016). Despite a range of government-funded public health campaigns, significant numbers of Australians continue to identify as smokers, a finding most marked amongst Indigenous and disadvantaged groups (Wiggington & Lee, 2012). Of particular concern to public health advocates has been the recent finding that many pregnant women, the long-term target of specific anti-smoking interventions, continue to report smoking behaviours. Indeed, national maternity indicators suggest that 1 in 7 Australian women smokes while pregnant, with prevalence higher among women who give birth in public hospitals, and those whose living contexts are rural and/or remote (Australian Institute of Health and Welfare, and National Perinatal Epidemiology and Statistics Unit, 2013).

In recent years, the widespread anti-smoking sentiment, and a burgeoning emphasis on a mother's responsibility to 'protect the health' of her foetus, have combined to position pregnant smokers as the object of particular censure. Within the discourse of the 'new public health', smoking in pregnancy is held to breach modern norms of 'reproductive citizenship' (Lupton, 2012) in which mothers are morally required to engage in healthy, risk-avoidant behaviours on behalf of their unborn child (Roy, 2008). As the surveillance and control of pregnant women's bodies has been normalised and naturalised, the conflation of 'healthy' and 'virtuous' behaviours has seen pregnant smokers experience judgement and confrontation in both private and public spheres (Bull, Burke, Walsh, & Whitehead, 2007). The notion that women are solely responsible (and, in the negative, culpable) for the health and development of their foetus has contributed to the increasing pressure placed upon them to quit smoking in order to conform to a 'good mother' ideal (Goodwin & Huppatz, 2010) now extended to women during pregnancy and even prior to conception (Fox, Nicolson, & Heffernan, 2009). Broader social inequities that may influence pregnant women's smoking and constrain cessation are absented in this dominant framework privileging an individualised account of health as impacted by 'virtue' and 'choice' (Gillies & Willig, 1997).

It is argued that the media play an important role in the dissemination and regulation of public understandings of health issues (Lyons, 2000) including pregnancy, motherhood, and 'risks' such as cigarette smoking. In news media contexts it is argued that the legitimacy afforded medical knowledge allows simplified, often moralising, 'scientific journalism' to define health issues as pressing social problems (Maher, Fraser, & Wright, 2010). With regard to smoking and pregnancy, this has been evident in foetal-centred accounts of mothers' 'failure to protect' their offspring from the documented harms of smoking exposure (Greaves, Cormier, Devries, Bottorff, & Abousaffy, 2003). While steeped in the language of rational empiricism, sensationalist reporting of scientific research in this area has served to define smoking in pregnancy as a problem requiring coercive intervention (Greaves & Poole, 2005). In more gossip-focused outlets, celebrity pregnancies have increasingly come under surveillance, with the bodies and behaviours of famous mothers-to-be documented for public consumption and judgement (Warin, Zivkovic, Moore, & Davies, 2012). In both 'informative' and 'gossip' platforms, it may be seen that the media wields considerable power in both determining, and policing, appropriate health behaviours in pregnancy (and those emblematic of 'good mothering').

In this paper, we examine a public account of smoking in pregnancy provided by a celebrity in the Australian mainstream media. Specifically, we focus on the way in which Chrissie Swan accounted, on radio, for her continued smoking while pregnant after photographic evidence of her behaviour entered the public domain.

Chrissie Swan's smoking 'confession'

Well-known and liked in Australia, Chrissie Swan's career began on reality television programme 'Big Brother' (2003). In 2010, Swan was a regular panel member on women's chat show 'The Circle', a role that saw her develop an identity as a humorous, down-to-earth mother of two. Chrissie's popular, relatable appeal led to her appointment in 2011 as host of the commercial drive-time radio programme 'The 3 pm Pickup' (a show marketed at women collecting their children from school), and as host of the television panel show 'Can of Worms' in 2012. In each of these roles, Chrissie's identity as a mother was paramount in the marketing and content of her broadcasts.

In 2013, 'Chrissie's radio confession' (as the transcript of her account of smoking while pregnant was entitled on the website of her radio network) received much subsequent media coverage (e.g. 'I knew it was wrong' Chrissie Swan admits to smoking while pregnant – The Sydney Morning Herald). In turn, this event and its aftermath led Swan to make further 'confessions' on radio, television and to the print media, prompting considerable public discussion around her behaviour and that of other pregnant smokers.

'Chrissie's confession' thus represents a unique context for the analysis of discourse around smoking in pregnancy. On one hand, Swan may be seen to represent an 'everymother', accounting for her smoking behaviour in a cultural context of zero tolerance. As previous qualitative research has indicated, women in this position have pervasively reported an awareness of social stigma (Bull et al., 2007; Wiggington

& Lee, 2012), feelings of guilt and shame (Nichter, Adrian, Goldade, Tesler, & Muramoto, 2008; Wood, France, Hunt, Eades, & Slack-Smith, 2008), and a requirement to deflect accusations of neglect (Irwin, Johnson, & Bottorff, 2005). In this sense, Swan may be understood as a woman positioned by public discourses of smoking as a breach of the risk-avoidant, 'unselfish nurturing' (Hays, 1996, p. x) inherent in the culturally approved ideal of modern motherhood (Lupton, 2011).

On the other hand, the public nature and dissemination of Swan's narrative suggests her 'confession' also represents a site in which cultural norms around smoking in pregnancy are being actively (re)produced. The compulsion to account publicly for her smoking bolsters the notion that this is an 'accountable issue', justifying and naturalising pregnant smokers as objects of public judgement and blame. In this sense, Swan's account may also be seen as part of the 'mediation' of health (Hodgetts, Bolam, & Stephens, 2005) through which taken-for-granted frameworks for understanding health concerns are defined, and approaches to addressing them legitimated, within dominant media narratives (Hodgetts & Chamberlain, 2006).

In analysing this situated example, we endeavour to examine the nature and consequences both of Chrissie's individual strategies of justification and sense-making about her smoking behaviour. In turn, we seek to analyse the broader implications of this public account in the reproduction and regulation of broader cultural understandings around smoking, pregnancy and health risks.

Method

The theoretical perspective of this paper is broadly social constructionist; our analysis is grounded in the assumption that talk reflects both the context in which it is generated, as well as broader patterns of collective understanding (Edley, 2001). As such, a synthetic approach to discourse analysis (Wetherell, 1998) is adopted, combining the traditions of conversation analysis and an interest in broader cultural and historical power relations. This approach to discourse analysis focuses on the 'action-orientation' of accounts (the notion that people use language to *do* things, e.g. justify, blame or persuade), holding that language is both constructed (from linguistic resources and rhetorical devices) and constructive (of identities, versions and realities).

More specifically, the analysis is concerned with the particular discursive practices that serve to explain Swan's smoking in pregnancy, and to manage her maternal identity in the context of her continued tobacco use. These explanations are considered within the broader discourse of the 'new public health' in which maternal 'management of risk' is a dominant sense-making framework.

For the purpose of analysis, audio of Swan's radio account was downloaded from the website of her broadcasting network (www.mix1011.com.au/shows/breakfast/listen/chrissies-confession) was transcribed verbatim, and is presented and analysed in order. In presenting the account, paragraph breaks reflect turns taken between Swan and co-presenters Jane Hall and Jamie Row (both of whom remained largely silent during the course of Swan's speech).

Analysis

'I just failed and failed'

From the outset of her radio broadcast, Swan's smoking in pregnancy is presented as an accountable issue (Wigginton & Lafrance, 2016).

> *Extract 1*:
>
> **Chrissie Swan (CS):**   This is a very big moment for me and I'm very nervous. Is it just me or did you have trouble giving up smoking when you were pregnant? That's right, I have a confession (cries) and that is that I have struggled terribly with totally giving up cigarettes since I found out that I was pregnant.
>
> **Jane Hall (JH):**   OK. That's alright.

CS: Up until about six years ago, I was what I would call a 'full time' smoker, I really gave it a nudge in um, in my twenties, as a lot of us did. [...] and then I got pregnant with Leo [Swan's first child] and I quit completely. For a couple of years, which was fantastic. Now sadly I picked it up again about a year ago but I was what I would call a 'not really' smoker. I never smoked at home and I never smoked around my family.

JH: It's alright.

CS: (Cries) I'd just sneak a few here and there and I know I'm not alone in this. Mainly I would do it in the car, in fact, I would only do it in the car when I was certain that I was alone. Then I found out six months ago that I was pregnant and it was a massive surprise and I tried to go cold turkey like I did with Leo and I was confident that I could do it. But I couldn't do it. And I just failed and failed. (Cries) Time after time. [...] Giving up is so hard, and I've really learned that in these last six months. These are not excuses, there are no excuses for smoking, absolutely none. I don't have one, I would, I would love to find one and I can't.

Throughout this extract, Swan draws upon, and naturalises, a foetal-centred account of the 'good mother'. Smoking, deemed relatively unproblematic in her younger, single years ('I really gave it a nudge in um, in my twenties'), is rendered inexcusable only at the point of impending motherhood with its attendant responsibility to put the health of children first. Swan's self-depiction as worthy of both praise for child-oriented quitting ('I got pregnant with Leo and I quit completely ... which was fantastic') and censure for failing to quit ('there are no excuses') positions women as fully responsible for the health (or otherwise) of their foetus at the expense of all other concerns. As Blum (2007) has argued, such accounts are grounded in a mother valour/mother blame binary in which failure to perform sanctioned maternal activities renders mothers more broadly responsible for the (poor) health outcomes of families, citizens and, ultimately, the nation.

Against this unequivocal account of maternal responsibility, Swan's continued smoking in pregnancy is positioned as a particularly contentious matter, and as a threat to her moral credibility. In turn, Swan provides what can be seen as an 'account' in this regard, a form of talk 'routinely expected whenever conduct falls outside the domain of normative expectations' (Arribas-Ayllon, Sarangi, & Clarke, 2008, p. 1522). More specifically, Swan draws upon three primary means of acknowledging the transgressive nature of her smoking behaviour (thus bolstering her identity as a 'good mother' who understands her responsibility to minimise foetal risk), while simultaneously managing a positive presentation of herself and her mothering.

At one level, Swan's account may be seen to emphasise the sustained effort she has put in to her attempts at smoking cessation. Extrematised representations (Pomerantz, 1986) of both the challenges she faced ('Giving up is so hard') and her repeated efforts to overcome them ('I just failed and failed ... Time after time') appear to assert the strongest case that she 'did her best' in anticipation of a potentially non-sympathetic hearing. Likewise, Swan emphasises her efforts towards harm reduction ('I never smoked at home and I never smoked around my family'; 'I'd just sneak a few here and there ... when I was certain that I was alone'), a strategy Wiggington and Lee (2012) have argued allows women to reposition themselves in a positive light and 'manage their "spoiled" identities as pregnant smokers' (p. 10). Finally, Swan makes an explicit acknowledgement of her guilt and shame in relation to her smoking ('there are no excuses for smoking, absolutely none'). This acknowledgement of transgression may also serve to align Swan with an audience inclined to be unsympathetic, the open sharing of guilt a means of shielding a speaker from the anticipated judgement of others (Irwin et al., 2005).

The account, therefore, may be seen to do a range of work to manage a positive identity for Swan in light of her 'confession'. At the same time, however, an orientation to pregnant women's 'natural' responsibility for managing foetal risk, and culpability when they fail to do so, may be seen to reproduce a particular version of the 'good mother', while cementing the issue of smoking in pregnancy as an issue of 'moral concern'. It may be argued that such a foetal-centred approach sidelines concern around a mother's *own* health in relation to smoking behaviours – a focus that may be of more utility in supporting family health in the longer term. Likewise, the mother blame/mother valour binary reproduced in such accounts may serve to support the more 'coercive, moralising' (Wiggington & Lee, 2012) flavour of anti-smoking interventions argued to disempower pregnant women during a period often characterised by an increased need for support (Greaves & Poole, 2005).

There's no 'right time to quit' when you're doing it all

After establishing an account of maternal responsibility for smoking cessation, Swan presents a narrative of the steps she took while endeavouring to quit.

Extract 2:

CS: … I'd win for a few days and then I would have a cigarette and I would feel terrible and wracked with guilt and then I'd be off the cigarettes for a week and then I'd get stressed out and I'd have one again.

[…]

When I realised I was having difficulty I went online and I looked for ways to quit and the first step, because you know I'm mad for Google

JH: God.

CS: The first step was find the right time to quit, that was step one. (Takes deep breath) And ordinarily that would be the easiest step of all, um, but at the time I was so busy and with so much on, I had two radio shows, Can of Worms had just started, a new TV show. Interstate travel every week, I had a weekly column, a relationship and a house to run, I was selling my house, I was trying to find somewhere else to live, I have a four year old as you know […] and there didn't seem to be any time at all, let alone the 'right time'. So I kept trying and falling down and the constant disappointment of feeling a failure had made me. (Sniff)

And I came up with a compromise with myself. It's so stupid but I made a deal. I would go easy on myself and smoke a few a week. Only when absolutely necessary, after work, alone, in the car and I figured it couldn't do any damage and it would let me deal with properly quitting when I wasn't so busy later on.

In Extract 2, smoking is presented as being a condition beyond Swan's volition, and as an (external-ised) compulsion she needed to 'fight' ('I'd win for a few days and then I'd have a cigarette'). In line with this medicalised framework, Swan presents her difficulty quitting as a health concern to be 'diagnosed' and 'treated'. After noting the problem, Swan explains that she immediately sought expert information as to the appropriate solution ('When I realised I was having difficulty I went online and I looked for ways to quit'). In turn, the notion that she found *the* answer ('the first step was to find the right time to quit') bolsters the status of smoking as a medical concern that, having been identified, may be treated by following sanctioned 'steps'.

The notion that quitting requires finding 'the right time' serves in the extract as a key means of managing Swan's accountability for her ongoing smoking behaviour, and locates the narrative within the context of a mother trying to 'do it all'. While presenting as someone who knew and accepted her responsibility to take steps towards quitting, her failure to quit is explained by external circumstances thwarting her efforts to take the requisite 'first step'. That Swan was busy 'doing it all' in both work and family spheres ('there didn't seem to be any time at all, let alone the "right time"') renders her failure to quit understandable, while reinforcing a 'supermum' positioning that would otherwise be undermined by her continued smoking behaviour. Against this background, Swan's harm minimisation efforts ('I would go easy on myself and smoke a few a week … it would let me deal with properly quitting when I wasn't so busy later on') appear similarly understandable, and potentially commendable. Likewise, her claim that 'it couldn't do any damage' represents a risk assessment that protects her from being positioned as deliberately harming her child.

As Hodgetts and Chamberlain (2006) have argued, media representations of health concerns such as smoking routinely frame these issues through a medical lens, focusing on lifestyle interventions with which individuals are 'morally required' to comply. In turn, they explain, attention to the socio-cultural factors that support and constrain health practices is regularly restricted. Yet, as the above extract illus-trates, it seems that a singular focus on women's 'responsibility to stop smoking' would deflect attention from the way in which the socio-cultural expectation that women 'do it all' may intersect with a medical discourse in a manner that serves to justify continued smoking. For Swan, the construction of smoking as a condition requiring action, coupled with the notion that a good mother 'does it all', suggests that the other factors constraining her quitting are also (solely) hers to manage. In turn, although external constraints to her quitting are identified, the location of the smoking problem squarely on Swan's shoulders may limit her capacity to access external supports.

Too hard to 'ask for help'

The notion that pregnant women bear singular responsibility for the health of their unborn children is pervasive throughout Swan's account, and is developed further in the extract below.

Extract 3:

CS: Well, two days ago a photographer followed me in my car after work and took a photo of me having that sneaky cigarette, it was my first for the week. I begged the photographers not to run the story because I know how bad it looks, it is bad.

JH: Mmm.

CS: And I also told them that it was a deeply shameful secret (Sniff) No one knew that I was having these five cigarettes a week. Not my mum, not my best friend, not my partner, not even you and Jamie.

JH: No.

CS: Because it's so, you know, the secret that is the most shameful is the hardest to ask for help about. (Sniff)

[…]

So I kept it all under wraps and dealt with it how I could, I felt that there was no one I could confess this to, no one I could say 'what can I do? This is hard for me – I was able to give up so easily with the others'. So I self-analysed and decided that this was the way I could get through it and keep the show on the road in terms of work and family commitments until the forced cold turkey of hospital. That was the plan.

In Extract 3, Swan presents an account of acute isolation in her efforts to quit smoking. Swan explains that those who might have been expected to serve as key social supports ('my mum, my best friend, my partner') remained unaware of her smoking because it was too shameful to confess ('the secret that is the most shameful is the hardest to ask for help about'). As was the case throughout the transcript, the shame around smoking depicted here arises from a construction of the behaviour as less 'unhealthy' than 'wrong' (Wiggington & Lee, 2012).

As a radio 'confession', Swan's account may be seen to be performing very specific identity work in terms of 'managing the message' with regard to her public persona. By aligning herself with potential critics of her behaviour ('I know how bad it looks. It is bad') and by arguably exaggerating her crime (it may be seen as overstatement to describe her 'five cigarettes a week' as a 'deeply shameful secret'), Swan may be seen to accept a vilified identity – an acceptance required to facilitate the public sympathy and forgiveness necessary for continued employment in the media (Wigginton & Lafrance, 2016).

Nonetheless, it may be argued that the discourse of good mothering Swan invokes – a discourse pervasive in public health messaging designed to encourage quitting behaviour (amongst other health behaviour change) – serves here to construct a direct impediment to smoking cessation. While Swan's account navigates a good mother position by orienting to guilt and shame at her failure to quit for her child, in the context of broader efforts to keep the family 'show on the road', the notion that such efforts might be reciprocal or supported is simultaneously undermined. Indeed, as this account suggests, the dual constructions of women as morally responsible for the health of their offspring, and as culpable for exposing them to risks, can engender a shame that may effectively constrains mothers' help-seeking options – potentially to considerable emotional and physical effect.

As Wiggington and Lee (2012, p. 11) have argued, social stigma around smoking in pregnancy can serve to 'marginalise smokers, creating a perceived need to present themselves dishonestly to others [which] may result in their avoiding contexts in which they may be offered support for cessation'. For someone in the public eye, and subject to community scrutiny, this is perhaps a particular concern for Swan ('I begged the photographers not to run the story because I know how bad it looks, it is bad'). Ultimately, as her account suggests, a socio-moral emphasis on a woman's responsibility for the health of her foetus – *at the expense* of a more broadly conceived social responsibility for the health of pregnant women – may serve to undermine efforts to address the 'problem' as it is dominantly defined.

The good mother versus the pregnant smoker – paradoxical accounting

Our analysis indicates that the relationship between conceptualisations of 'good motherhood' and smoking during pregnancy is paradoxical. If it is shameful for a mother to smoke (because a good mother would protect her foetus), how can she ask for the help she may need to quit and 'put her foetus first'? Likewise, if a discourse of addiction is dominant (and relies on a construction of the mother as responsible for fighting the problem), how easy is it to acquire the support she may need to find the 'right time' to begin?

As Warin et al. (2012) have argued, constructions of exclusive maternal responsibility for foetal health not only limit the scope of risk management 'problems', but likewise narrow options for their solution. In the case of smoking in pregnancy, this focus on a woman's 'moral responsibility to quit for her child' may undermine mothers' capacity to embark upon, and sustain, quitting behaviours over the long term – behaviours that must be understood in the context of a range of socio-cultural expectations around 'good motherhood' by which pregnant women are simultaneously positioned.

'I know it's wrong, it's madness' – an illustration of paradoxical accounting

The paradoxical nature of identity management for pregnant smokers is illustrated in the final extract, below.

Extract 4:

CS: And here's the truth. Obviously I know it is wrong, I'm not an idiot. No smoker wants to smoke, especially when they are pregnant but it is clearly an addiction and a very serious one because it can cloud your judgement and can make the unthinkable somehow ok (deep breath). As a listener to this show, you know I am devoted to my children (deep breath).

I would never do anything to harm them (sniff). And yet here I am, having five cigarettes a week and justifying it, it's madness (sniff).

I cannot explain it. I knew it was wrong but there's so much terrible judgement that only awful people and bad parents and idiots and bogans smoke during pregnancy and I didn't feel like I belonged in any of those categories (sniff).

In Extract 4, Swan externalises and personifies addiction, an account that once again enables her to present as a 'good but thwarted' mother. As we have outlined above, the medicalised, addiction discourse positions cigarette smoking as a problem to be treated via specific, sanctioned steps and limits responsibility for taking them to the pregnant mother alone. In this extract, however, the addiction discourse serves another function in justifying Swan's continued smoking: addiction is depicted as undermining her very capacity to make the 'right decision' to quit.

Throughout the extract, the language of cognition dominates. Addiction is depicted actively as a force that can 'cloud your judgement' and 'make the unthinkable somehow ok'. Ultimately, this serves to offer resolution to the identity paradox faced by a mother who would not 'do anything to harm' her children, but continues to justify having 'five cigarettes a week'. In the context of her narrative, perhaps only an account of irrationality ('It's madness') could satisfactorily explain why a mother who knows 'it is wrong' and is 'not an idiot' would continue to smoke during pregnancy. Swan's self-presentation as distinct from 'idiots' and 'bogans' – inference-rich categories whose members who might normatively be expected to smoke thoughtlessly or wilfully in pregnancy (Bayer & Colgrove, 2002) – also bolsters her 'good mother' position: she is neither thoughtless nor wilful but constrained by an addiction that limits her capacity to put good motives into action.

The concept of rationality is argued to be at the heart of public health interventions in the area of smoking, and more broadly. Grounded in models of social cognition, many health promotion campaigns assume that individuals undertake conscious analyses of health risks, thus impacting their mental representations of health issues and sparking behaviour change (Horrocks & Johnson, 2014). Anti-smoking campaigns, in particular, are pervasively predicated on the notion that a rational decision-maker, provided with information about the risks of smoking, will change their beliefs and attitudes and be inclined to quit (Gillies & Willig, 1997).

In the context of Swan's account, it seems that the notion of 'rationality' with regard to smoking in pregnancy may be more usefully interrogated than assumed. Here, it is hard to maintain a sense that cognitive factors are the most important determinants of behaviour change when rationality is routinely undermined in favour of an 'irrationality' account that allows the continuation of a 'good mother' position.

In light of these complexities, it seems that anti-smoking interventions that focus on information provision, assuming a rational decision-maker, may be of less utility than an approach addressing the range of social and cultural factors by which pregnant mothers' smoking identities (and subsequent behaviours) are constrained. Indeed, it seems that the dominance of the 'ir/rationality' concept in public health anti-smoking discourse may, paradoxically, intersect with conceptualisations of 'addiction' in a manner that may discursively limit options for sense-making – and action – with regard to behaviour change.

Conclusion

In recent years, tobacco-related public health interventions have been dominantly informed by addiction and lifestyle models, the result of which, as Poland et al. (2006:59) argue, has been to underplay the 'social meaning of smoking in … people's everyday lives'. In the context of maternal smoking, the deflection of attention from social constructions of 'good mothering', and the concomitant expectation that mothers manage the 'risk, danger, responsibility' (Lupton, 2011) of foetal well-being seems a particularly significant omission.

Our analysis suggests that while accounts of maternal responsibility ostensibly encourage quitting behaviours on the grounds of 'protecting the foetus', they can also serve to justify and explain continued smoking in pregnancy. As Swan's account illustrates, reproduction of the notion that a child's health is 'the mother's concern' may serve to constrain responsibility for smoking cessation to women, limiting the scope of the 'problem' rather than expanding it to include a focus on the potential contributions of partners and other supporters. Likewise, such accounts may serve to sideline concern around a pregnant woman's *own* health, and the support needs (social, economic, domestic) that may be required to help her quit.

In broader terms, constructions of women as 'accountable' for foetal health reproduce understandings of smoking in pregnancy as a pressing moral issue. In line with messages of the new public health that define health-promoting behaviours as 'moral obligation', this construction serves to position women as ethically required to manage risks such as cigarette smoking. In turn, as Lupton (2012) has argued, women who do not adhere to this modern norm of reproductive citizenship become subject to public censure.

In the case of Swan's 'confession', it must be noted that constructions of maternal smoking were mobilised within a specific rhetorical context: a public broadcast arguably designed to assuage a potentially critical audience. Nonetheless, Swan's account of her 'shame' at breaching the norms of 'good motherhood' both draws upon and reproduces what Wigginton and Lafrance (2016) describe as the 'discursive silencing' of pregnant smokers. By aligning her account with the only 'hearable' story of smoking (it is 'bad', 'inexcusable', a 'failure'), Swan positions pregnant smokers as having relinquished any moral authority to speak, and make sense of, their experience. In turn, her account may be seen to bolster a discursive silencing that renders women's smoking behaviours 'untellable' (Wigginton & Lafrance, 2016), thereby limiting their capacity to be open in seeking the informational and social resources needed to help them quit.

In Swan's account, the contrasting imperatives that a mother 'acknowledge that she should not smoke' while (responsibly) admitting to continued smoking ultimately serves to privilege an addiction discourse in which an inherent 'irrationality' explains otherwise inexplicable behaviour. The identity paradox ('I know it's wrong … yet here I am having five cigarettes a week') is resolved through a construction of 'good intentions thwarted' by an irrational addiction (largely) beyond her control. In turn, while a positive identity is managed, the broader effect of such an account is once again to medicalise smoking in a manner that deflects attention from the social, cultural and economic factors that influence smoking behaviours.

As a media broadcast, the public nature of Swan's 'confession' means that her account of smoking in pregnancy becomes implicated in the constitution of taken-for-granted frameworks for understanding this issue, and the legitimation of specific approaches by which it should be addressed (Hodgetts and Chamberlain (2006). Indeed, it seems the sense-making framework Swan develops serves to justify the kind of moralising intervention arguably exemplified in the Australian Government's current 'Quit for you, quit for two' intervention, in which the importance of quitting smoking in pregnancy is underlined via reference to women's singular responsibility (e.g. 'When you smoke, she gets less oxygen'). Yet, as our analysis suggests, an exclusive campaign focus on information provision (with a view to emphasising women's moral accountability) may be less fruitful than a focus on *broadening* responsibility for maternal and foetal health to include partners, extended families and communities. Insights may be usefully drawn from recent public health breastfeeding campaigns such as UNICEF's *Why breastfeeding mums deserve our support* (underpinned by the tagline 'Good for bubs, good for mums, good for us all') which emphasises both the benefits for, and responsibilities of, communities that prioritise both maternal and foetal health.

Disclosure statement

No potential conflict of interest was reported by the authors.

References

Arribas-Ayllon, M., Sarangi, S., & Clarke, A. (2008). Managing self responsibility through other-oriented blame: Family accounts of genetic testing. *Social Science and Medicine, 66*, 1521–1532.

Australian Institute of Health and Welfare, and National Perinatal Epidemiology and Statistics Unit. (2013). *National core maternity indicators* (Cat, no. PER 58). Canberra: AIHW.

Bayer, R., & Colgrove, J. (2002). Science, politics, and ideology in the campaign against environmental tobacco smoke. *American Journal of Public Health, 92*, 949–954.

Blum, L. (2007). Mother-blame in the Prozac nation: Raising kids with invisible disabilities. *Gender & Society, 21*, 202–226.

Bull, L., Burke, R., Walsh, S., & Whitehead, E. (2007). Social attitudes towards smoking in pregnancy in East Surrey: A qualitative study of smokers, former smokers and non-smokers. *Journal of Neonatal Nursing, 13*, 100–106.

Edley, N. (2001). Analysing masculinity: Interpretative repertoires, subject positions and ideological dilemmas. In M. Wetherell, S. Taylor, & S. J. Yates (Eds.), *Discourse as data: A guide to analysis* (pp. 189–229). London: Sage.

Fox, R., Nicolson, P., & Heffernan, K. (2009). Pregnancy police? Maternal bodies, pregnancy and food. In P. Jackson (Ed.), *Changing families, changing food* (pp. 57–74). Basingstoke: Palgrave Macmillan.

Gillies, V., & Willig, C. (1997). 'You get the nicotine and that in your blood' – Constructions of addiction and control in women's accounts of cigarette smoking. *Journal of Community & Applied Social Psychology, 7*, 285–301.

Goodwin, S., & Huppatz, K. (2010). *The good mother: Contemporary motherhood in Australia.* Sydney: Sydney University Press.

Greaves, L., & Poole, N. (2005). Victimized or validated? Responses to substance-using pregnant women. *Canadian Woman Studies, 24*, 87–92.

Greaves, L., Cormier, R., Devries, K., Bottorff, J., & Abousaffy, D. (2003). *Expecting to quit: A best practices review of smoking cessation interventions for pregnant and postpartum girls and women.* Vancouver: British Columbia Centre for Excellence for Women's Health.

Hays, S. (1996). *The cultural contradictions of motherhood.* New Haven, CT: Yale University Press.

Hodgetts, D., & Chamberlain, K. (2006). Developing a critical media research agenda for health psychology. *Journal of Health Psychology, 11*, 317–327.

Hodgetts, D., Bolam, B., & Stephens, C. (2005). Mediation and the construction of contemporary understandings of health and lifestyle. *Journal of Health Psychology, 10*, 123–136.

Horrocks, C., & Johnson, S. (2014). A socially situated approach to inform ways to improve health and welbeing. *Sociology of Health and Illness, 36*, 175–186.

Irwin, L., Johnson, J., & Bottorff, J. (2005). Mothers who smoke: Confessions and justifications. *Health Care for Women International, 26*, 557–590.

Lupton, D. (2011). 'The best thing for the baby': Mothers' concepts and experiences related to promoting their infants' health and development. *Health, Risk & Society, 13*, 637–651.

Lupton, D. (2012). 'Precious cargo': Foetal subjects, risk and reproductive citizenship. *Critical Public Health, 22*, 329–340.

Lyons, A. (2000). Examining media representations: Benefits for health psychology. *Journal of Health Psychology, 5*, 349–358.

Maher, J., Fraser, S., & Wright, J. (2010). Framing the mother: Childhood obesity, maternal responsibility and care. *Journal of Gender Studies, 19*, 233–247.

Nichter, M., Adrian, S., Goldade, K., Tesler, L., & Muramoto, M. (2008). Smoking and harm-reduction efforts among postpartum women. *Qualitative Health Research, 18*, 1184–1194.

Poland, B., Frohlich, K., Haines, R. J., Mykhalovskiy, E., Rock, M., & Sparks, R. (2006). The social context of smoking: The next frontier in tobacco control? *Tobacco Control, 15*, 59–63.

Pomerantz, A. (1986). Extreme case formulations: A way of legitimizing claims. *Human Studies, 9*, 219–229.

Roy, S. (2008). 'Taking charge of your health': Discourses of responsibility in English-Canadian women's magazines. *Sociology of Health & Illness, 30*, 463–477.

Warin, M., Zivkovic, T., Moore, V., & Davies, M. (2012). Mothers as smoking guns: Fetal overnutrition and the reproduction of obesity. *Feminism & Psychology, 22*, 360–375.

Weiland, T., Jelinek, G., Taylor, S., & Taylor, D. (2016). Tobacco smoking by adult emergency department patients in Australia: A point-prevalence study. *Public Health Research Practice, 26*(3), e2631634.

Wetherell, M. (1998). Positioning and interpretative repertoires: Conversation analysis and post-structuralism in dialogue. *Discourse & Society, 9*, 387–412.

Wigginton, B. & Lafrance, M. N. (2016). How do women manage the spoiled identity of a 'pregnant smoker'? An analysis of discursive silencing in women's accounts. *Feminism & Psychology, 26*, 30–51.

Wiggington, B., & Lee, C. (2012). A story of stigma: Australian women's accounts of smoking during pregnancy. *Critical Public Health, 23*(4), 1–16.

Wood, L., France, K., Hunt, K., Eades, S., & Slack-Smith, L. (2008). Indigenous women and smoking during pregnancy: Knowledge, cultural contexts and barriers to cessation. *Social Science & Medicine, 66*, 2378–2389.

8 Perception and translation of numbers

The case of a health campaign in Denmark

Dorthe Brogård Kristensen, Charlotte Bredahl Jacobsen and Signe Pihl-Thingvad

ABSTRACT

This article explores the translation of numeric health communications from the authorities to ordinary citizens. Based on qualitative interviews and document analysis, it follows the life of a Danish health campaign called '6 a day' from its initiation to its dissemination, and finally to its place in the perceptions and health practices of citizens. While the definition of the target of '6 a day' was clearly anchored in social and scientific contexts, it incorporated considerable ambiguity and scientific uncertainty, flaws which were deliberately kept from citizens. The number '6' was meant to appear unquestionable. We suggest that this way of making and disseminating numeric health campaigns may best be understood as a process of creating a mould and offering it to citizens to fill with their own health practices. Such a process is rife with translations and the article analyses both these and their impact on citizens' health practices and perceptions. We conclude that the success of the campaign lies in its implicit logic and the agency it fosters, rather than its ability to improve health literacy or make citizens aspire to specific health targets. The article thereby contributes to an understanding of the effects of numeric health communications. Health communicators may also gain from an increased awareness of the processes of translation involved in health messages created as moulds.

Introduction

In a number of situations, citizens are expected (and expect) to receive information and adapt their practices according to the advice offered by the health authorities. In many cases, health communications have been conveyed using numbers so that citizens may quickly understand and act upon them: for instance, '5 a day' or 'Walk 10,000 steps a day'. This information may be simple and easy to remember and follow, but it remains unexplored whether the use of numbers in such communications enables citizens to make informed health decisions. Against this background, the focus of this article is on how numbers in public health campaigns are translated from the public domain into the everyday practices of citizens. How are they perceived, given meaning, and embodied in people's health practices? We explore the use of numbers in two parallel contexts – the making of public health campaigns and their interpretation by the target audience – in order to describe the processes by which a health campaign constructs and mobilizes specific health practices. More specifically, we explore the design, dissemination and perceptions of a Danish health campaign that was known as '6 a day' (*6 om dagen*). Inspired by

Actor Network Theory, the focus is on how this specific campaign was translated into everyday practice and perceptions by stakeholders and citizens. We show that, while the use of numbers provides a certain legitimacy and a logic of self-discipline, numbers are understood differently and reshaped in new embodiments or instantiations. The campaign serves to shape the structure of people's practices by referring to a specific logic, but in a way that also fosters a sense of creativity and agency.

'6 a day' as a mould

The slogan '6 a day – eat more fruit and vegetables' was launched as a public-private partnership between a range of health authorities, nongovernmental organizations and private trade associations. Utilizing the concept of translation we follow the life of the campaign as we conduct an analysis focusing on the translation of meanings of the message '6 a day' as it travels from the health authorities to citizens. According to Callon (2007) translation is the mechanism by which the social and natural world progressively takes form. When a phenomenon moves from one sphere (it may be the sphere in which it originated) to another, a translation process takes place during which the phenomenon, in this case the message, is endowed with a different meaning which may simplify the original version, while at the same time creating uncertainties and ambiguities.

In this case, the message of the campaign was communicated through a numerical logic. We therefore regard numbers as actants that are translated from one social context to another, analysis of which may take place by tracing their roots, pursuing their meanings and analysing them as phenomena that have an impact upon the relations of which they are a part (Latour, 1991). This perspective provides a tool to explore how numbers translate from public authorities to citizens. We will show how actors involved in the Danish health campaign created the message '6 a day' in a way that may best be understood as a work of constructing a mould, and then offering the hollow form to the public. Understanding the message '6 a day' as a mould makes it possible to grasp important characteristics of these kinds of health campaigns and their translations. Our argument is that a mould produces a particular semantic form that makes it easier for a health message to travel across different spheres (from public authorities to citizens); it shapes the structure of people's practices by referring to a specific logic, but in a way that fosters a sense of creativity and agency. To illustrate the concept of the mould, we may imagine a hollow form. A long process is required to create a mould, and knowledge and various logics – or networks of meaning – are used to build its exact form. When the form is complete, the inner material that was used to create it is removed and an empty semantic mould remains – ready for the creation of new figures. A significant amount of knowledge and research on health was used to build the mould '6 a day'; however, as the message was disseminated to the public, this knowledge was deliberately not communicated. Instead, the public received an empty mould with which to form and shape their own health practices (Figure 1).

Logics inherent in the use of numbers

In this article, we build on the work of scholars who have studied the logics inherent in the use of numbers in western societies. Their research points to the processes through which numbers become attractive means of communication to the authorities as well as to ordinary citizens. As argued by Poovey (1998), since the seventeenth century, technologies of measurement have been used as tools to produce legitimacy and authority. The production of systematic knowledge has influenced government practices in the use of numerical representation as the preferred mode for generating useful facts. Other scholars have dealt with standardization as a process of constructing uniformities across time and space that may function as an alternative to expert authority (Timmerman & Epstein, 2010, p. 71). Such standardization fuelled the growth of scientists' authority (Porter, 1995) and the 'infrastructural' power of the modern state (Timmerman & Epstein, 2010).

Thus, various scholars have pointed out that numbers appeal to governmental bodies because they communicate in a certain manner. For example, numbers can give the impression of being exact and based on scientific research, qualities that make them suitable for communicating a kind of absolutism in public life (Porter, 1995). At the same time, numbers also allow for flexibility in the content of a specific message. Discussing the processes that enable quantified knowledge to be so extraordinarily flexible that any issue can be formulated using the language of numbers – permitting reasoning to become more uniform and to appear more rigorous – Roy Porter writes:

> The appeal of numbers is especially compelling to bureaucratic officials who lack the mandate of a popular election or divine right. Arbitrariness and bias are the most usual ground upon which officials are criticized. A decision made by numbers (or by explicit rules of some other sort) has at least the appearance of being fair and impersonal. (Porter, 1995, p. 8)

In this way, public authorities can use the number to communicate an 'objective message', disguising any underlying ambiguities and subjective or political biases the message may contain, while at the same time allowing citizens to interpret the numbers in different ways, thereby reducing the risk of communicating unpopular political messages.

While there is considerable literature on the use by the authorities of calculative practices, the role played by numbers in the everyday health practices of citizens has not been extensively covered (Lupton, 2013), although there are some findings relevant for our attempt to understand this sphere. Miller (2004, p. 179) analyses the work of calculation and describes how accounting practices can generally be regarded as 'technologies of government' as they shape and transform human organization. He links calculative practices with values such as individual responsibility and self-regulation, and argues that both the language and the practice of calculation have become part of everyday life. Through technologies of quantification certain events are made visible and can then become viable objects of modulation and transformation (Miller, 2004). A Danish study by Oxlund (2012) provides an empirical example of this, arguing that representations of numbers in elderly people's narratives about their health and illness indicate that such references have not only entered citizens' language, but also their ontologies. Oxlund talks of an emergent numeric ontology that informs our bodies, the organization of our health care system, and the shape of our health care technologies (Mol, 2002).

Another branch of literature that provides a deeper understanding of this discussion is that pertaining to the quantified self and self-tracking (e.g. Lupton, 2013; Nafus & Sherman, 2014; Pantzer & Ruckenstein, 2015; Sharon & Zandbergen, 2016), which clarifies how the logics inherent in numbers appeal to ordinary citizens. While some of these researchers have discussed the disciplining power of self-quantification along much the same lines as Miller (Lupton, 2013), others have highlighted the fact that self-tracking by means of visualization can produce concrete data that function as a window *into* the self and a mirror *of* the self (Nafus & Sherman, 2014). The numerical data output and visualizations produced by wearables and apps are internalized and also used as a way of understanding personal identity by the individual citizen; yet the numbers also serve as an objective externalization that is perceived as free from human influence and bias, and can be used by the individual to communicate self-identity in a more objective way. Lomborg and Frandsen (2015) add to our understanding by looking into the communicative properties of self tracking. They argue that self-tracking and quantifying the resulting data offer together effective communicative tools for people which they can use to communicate in a simple way with the system, the self, and their peers (Lomborg & Frandsen, 2015).

It is striking how the objective gaze created by numbers seems as appealing to citizens' health practices at an individual level as it does to public authorities aiming to shape health practices on a population level. Both individual citizens and public authorities draw on a specific inherent logic in numbers that facilitates the communication of health messages. In summary, using numbers to communicate provides a simple, objective, authoritative and legitimate tool for sending messages about health practices. In the following, we connect these insights from the literature on the use of numbers by public authorities and citizens to analyse the parallel processes taking place as the '6 a day' campaign was developed, disseminated, and taken up by ordinary citizens.

Methods

In order to analyse how the public authorities constructed the '6 a day' health message as a mould in the campaign to generate specific health practices among Danish citizens, we used qualitative methodology; this centres on empirical descriptions and analyses of the processes taking place, thereby unravelling the ways in which the message and its truth were constructed in its specific context. We focused on the creation and mobilization of different interests in the translation process from the sender (the Danish Health authorities and the private companies using the campaign) to the receiver (Danish citizens), following the history of the message and observing its influence on citizens' health practices. To that end, we applied several methods of data collection: (I) Six individual semi-structured interviews – with experts from the public health authorities and nongovernmental health organizations who developed and implemented the campaign – in which interviewees were given the opportunity to tell their stories of the making of the campaign, their own involvement, and their reflections; (II) four individual semi-structured interviews with food companies that assisted in implementing the campaign, in which the representatives were invited to reflect upon their interests and role; (III) analysis of scientific reports of dietary recommendations, market analysis, and marketing documents related to the campaign in order to scrutinize the creation and implementation of the campaign; (IV) participant observation and walk-alongs (Kusenbach, 2003) in supermarkets with 20 citizens focusing on the use of public health messages in their 'decoding' of brands, logos, and food declarations; and (V) 12 in-depth interviews with selected people from the walk-alongs in which they were invited to talk freely about their perceptions and practices related to food consumption and health.

All the interviews were transcribed and coded. We used a meta-matrix (Miles, Huberman, & Saldaña, 2014, p. 135) to search for logics and mechanisms in the construction, enactment and perception of numbers in the different stages of the translation process. We looked for what was present and what was absent in the data (Law, 2004), where data seemed thick and well connected to massive networks of meaning, and where the opposite was the case (Geertz, 1973).

The case: '6 a day'

The slogan '6 a day – eat more fruit and vegetables' was launched in 1998. The bodies who took part in the first phase of the campaign were the Danish Veterinary and Food Administration, the Danish Fruit, Vegetable, and Potato Board, the Danish Agriculture and Food Council, Danish Horticulture, the Danish Heart Foundation, the Danish Cancer Society, and the Danish Health Authority. Private companies were also invited to join the campaign as partners. The partners each contributed DKK 150,000 (equivalent to around 22,000 USD) to the campaign and were then free to use the logo in relevant activities. Subsequently it has appeared in cook books, on juice cartons and packages of fruit and vegetables, in campaigns by the Danish Cancer Society, and so forth.

The campaign '6 a day' consists of a logo with the simple message that everyone should consume six pieces of fruit and vegetables per day. The campaign was owned by the partnership and aimed at generating initiatives encouraging Danes to make dietary changes that included fruit and vegetable subscription schemes in schools, surveys of consumers' attitudes to frozen and processed fruit and vegetables, and attempts to introduce more fruit and vegetables in canteens in schools and at work places. In August 2002, the '6 a day' campaign won the Columbus Egg prize, awarded by the advertising industry in recognition of 'an outstanding example of the fact that a broad cooperation between interested parties in both the private and public sectors is the way forward in the long, tough haul of changing attitudes and modifying behaviour'. Overall, the campaign has been perceived as one of the most successful ever in Denmark, due to its wide recognition.[1]

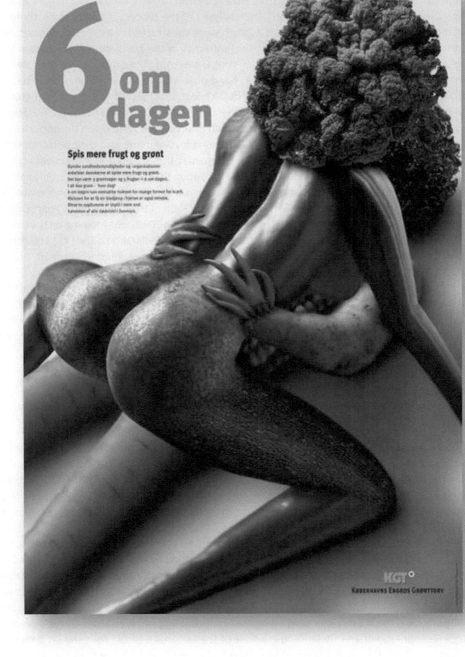

Figure 1. The poster '6 a day'.

Construction of the mould '6 a day'

We begin our analysis of the campaign, which marked a change in Danish health campaigns, by examining the logic of negotiations taking place among the partners. Up until '6 a day' was launched, health communications had been shaped by an approach whose principal goals were providing competence, inspiration, and ideas to the public connected with how to eat healthier food. '6 a day' was different, being more grounded in the natural sciences by the addition of clinical research. In addition it had a new focus on concrete messages and on 'availability', that is, on structural prevention combined with attention to communicative strategies, partnership and story-making. According to experts from the public authorities, the aim of the campaign was to make an impact on the whole of society, while the prime actors were not individual citizens, but institutional actors: the school canteens, workplaces, and supermarkets that would ensure that healthy eating became a more common and automatic choice among citizens.

Accordingly, many of the experts who were interviewed had relatively few thoughts about how the campaign would reach the citizens and affect their approach to healthy eating habits. On the other hand, they could all offer elaborate accounts of their involvement with, and considerations about, the interests and needs of institutional actors and private stakeholders. Thus, in the first phase of designing the campaign, the citizens as receivers were not in focus, and there were no intentional strategies directed at how the campaign should affect citizens' practices. Instead, all the experts interviewed emphasized the cooperation and trust between the public and private participants, their common work on structural availability, and their consensus never to challenge the recommendation (6 a day) in public but, rather, to leave room for interpretation of how people might follow it. Thus, from early on the partners were very careful to construct a single and clear message, but one which did not convey specific actions or practices. As such, the message in the campaign was intentionally created as a hollow semantic form – a mould – that left room for interpretation and agency on the part of its target audience.

The construction of '6 a day'

The campaign was inspired by global trends of encouraging citizens to increase their consumption of fruits and vegetables. At the same time, the intention of the authorities was to build a campaign based on scientific evidence. To do so, two commissions were established: one working on the basis of scientific evidence and the other working with communication strategies. The first group developed a report that could support the recommendation of the consumption of certain quantities of fruit and vegetables with scientific evidence. It documented a correlation between type two diabetes, obesity, cardio vascular diseases, and certain types of cancer, and the low consumption of fruits and vegetables (Trolle, Fagt, & Ovesen, 1998); however, while the report observed that diet played a significant role, the precise effect was not documented. It concluded with the assertion:

A daily intake of about 600 grams of fruit and vegetables in adults might be associated with lower risk of occurrence of ischemic heart disease and a number of important cancers. The intake of fruit and vegetables should be increased – preferably up to a daily amount of about 600 gram or more. (Trolle, Fagt, & Ovesen, 1998, p. 13)

When interviewed, the founder of the campaign, Morten Meyer Strunge, pointed out, 'Now, if you analyse this conclusion, you will realize that it holds a reservation in every sentence.' In other words, the scientific commission could not provide the campaign with a clear and single rule to follow. Strunge was inspired by the US campaign '5 a Day', supported by a scientific review process, which has also been used in the UK, Germany, Spain and Chile, later replaced in the US with the slogan 'Fruits & Veggies – More Matters'. In Argentina and the Netherlands the slogan '2 + 2 veggies and fruits' was used while Australia has opted for a 'Go for 2 & 5' campaign (Anker, Kristensen, & Brennan, 2015). Thus, while several campaigns make reference to a target number, these numbers fluctuate from country to country. Still, Strunge found it important that the Danish campaign, parallel to other national campaigns, used a single number to transfer the health message.

The interviews revealed that other experts from the health authorities were sceptical about the use of numbers, however, and especially the number 'six', as they were concerned with social inequalities and wanted to provide a message that did not seem unrealistic; six pieces per day seemed to be too high to be an attainable goal for many citizens. The interviews exposed a series of pragmatic attempts to reach consensus, as the scientific evidence was not sufficiently solid to claim that exactly 600 grams a day would produce the best diet for all, and there was also significant ambiguity in the message that should be addressed. For example, would the six a day include potatoes? Or did people already eat so many potatoes that it was better to exclude potatoes to secure variety? Should it be '6 a day' or '600 grams a day'? Should it be communicated as an interval, or was an exact number a better form of communication? And, after all, how significant is the effect on lowering the risk of lifestyle-related illnesses? These ambiguities resulted in a shift in focus in the negotiations related to the construction of the message from in-depth scientific discussions to how the involved partners could make the message appear trustworthy and appealing.

With input from the communication experts the final recommended number was chosen as six, which in Danish has a double significance, also meaning sex. This was not a crucial point in the partners' coming to the decision, but they all agreed it gave the campaign a humorous twist which made it easier to communicate. Furthermore, the partners were concerned about avoiding a paternalistic tone in the communication. The main aim was to find a message that was easily understood, and it was feared that a lack of clarity could cloud interest and curiosity (Trolle, Fagt, & Ovesen, 1998, p. 181).

The benefit of the pragmatic solutions agreed upon by both the health authorities and the food industry was that it became possible to engage in a joint effort to make the brand visible and to increase accessibility. The partners made an agreement not to use the campaign's sexual allusion explicitly, while also acknowledging that the number six could be understood in different ways. Despite the fact that there was some protest against the '6 a day' campaign, on the basis that it was an overly simplified message that could easily cause confusion and had excessively strong 'sexual associations' (Trolle, Fagt, & Ovesen, 1998, p. 194), the group eventually decided on '6 a day' based on the pragmatic arguments discussed above. This construction process shows that while the number might stand as a neutral scientific entity in many campaigns, it is in fact a historical construct, influenced by negotiations among the involved actors, and affected by more general global power relations (Miller, 2004). In the Danish campaign both scientific and pragmatic arguments were used to create the final message and decide on '6 a day'; however, ultimately, pragmatic reasoning was dominant in the process.

The translation of '6 a day' among Danish citizens

Despite the in-depth discussions and data-based research by the partners involved in designing the campaign, the scientific evidence behind the campaign was never communicated to the public. This confirms Latour's (1999) argument that science constructs artificial entities of knowledge that stand as units while the context in which they are produced is often rendered invisible. In a similar vein, Miller points to the interesting fact that even while accounting and calculations affect the social reality in which we live, including the way we assess methods of maintaining the nation's health and education, the calculative practice involved is often invisible to the public (Miller, 2004). This is a very accurate description of the translation process in this case. Once the standard '6 a day' was established, the work required to make it possible, as well as the ambiguity and pragmatic thinking that accompanied the final decisions, was made invisible (see also Timmerman & Epstein, 2010, p. 83). Hence, '6 a day' became a hollow mould for the translation of the health message to the citizens.

A translation process from one sphere to another involves changes and displacements in the phenomenon being transferred – in this case the message '6 a day'. Citizens' perception of the campaign's message was not a focus during the designing phase, but this aspect of the campaign became more salient when private companies took up the logo. In this process, a new translation took place which was grounded in the companies' needs to sell their products. Although the original partners had agreed not to use sexual undertones in the campaign, they were unable to control the message in the hands of commercial agents. A poster was produced by a private company (Grønttorvet) in which sexuality was an explicit feature, communicated by an image of vegetables having sex. In the public sphere, this poster became a hallmark of the campaign, and it is still displayed in some grocery shops today.

Hence, the translation process continued after the partners involved in designing the campaign had reached an agreement on the specific message. Today, the campaign is well-known by most Danes and associated strongly with its sexual innuendo. Recently, the campaign has been taken over by a private organization for agriculture and food,[2] relaunched with a more explicit reference to the double meaning of six, and renamed 'the fifty shades of vegetables'.

Thus, it was the poster that made the campaign highly salient in the public sphere. All the citizens in our study recalled the poster with the vegetables simulating sex and, to varying degrees, paid attention to the message. It is worth noting, however, that the basic structure and numerical logic of the mould was not transformed in this translation process, as using a number for management of food consumption was never questioned. On the other hand, the stand-alone number (six) left open a space for creativity and agency. In the following, we will examine more closely how citizens perceived the numerical logic offered by the mould '6 a day' and how it influenced their health practices.

Citizens' perceptions of the number in the campaign

It is tempting to conclude from the interviews that the citizens did not make much sense of the number six at all. Most informants showed a relaxed attitude towards the number as a target, but generally believed that they ought to eat more fruits and vegetables. The perception was that the campaign did not communicate any new knowledge; consequently, most of the informants interpreted the message to the effect that the exact number did not matter. Hence, the initiators' pragmatic approach to the figure was to some extent shared by the citizens, though based on other rationales. Some did not pay it significant attention because they found it a difficult target, some thinking that '6 a day' meant eating six portions of fruit (not vegetables), only noticing the first part of the message's tag; they had heard that it was not healthy to eat so much fruit due to the high sugar content of some of them. When asked about the importance of eating fruits and vegetables, few could point to any specific health benefits, rather voicing a general ideas that it increases 'healthiness', that 'greens contain vitamins', and that it is good for 'keeping the engine going'. Hence, people did not 'fill' the hollow mould with scientific evidence about the benefits of eating fruit and vegetables. It was clear that they did not share knowledge of this kind with the initiators of the campaign. Hence, whereas the pragmatic stance of the initiators was related to the *uncertainty* of the scientific evidence, the pragmatic stance of citizens appeared more the consequence of the hollowness of the mould and citizens' own responsibility of filling it with relevant health knowledge and practices.

Nonetheless, despite their pragmatic attitude, the number still mattered to informants in terms of communicating a certain logic. Bente, a 35-year-old mother, related to '6 a day' as a moral rule, using it to discipline herself in her choices of food. Even though she did not adhere to the exact number of fruit and vegetables, she perceived the message as an objective truth – a recommendation that should be followed. Bente commented that she trusted the message and did not question how the policy-makers arrived at their conclusions, believing that those responsible 'did a good job', and adding that 'as long as rules are realistic, no one poses any questions'. This way of thinking was mirrored by Annette – a woman aged 67 – who remarked: 'Those experts, they have to know why it is exactly six pieces.' At the same time, neither of the two women took the number too literally. As Bente remarked, 'As a woman, I do know that it is healthier to choose an apple or a carrot over a cream puff. I think we just need to rely on our common sense.' While the informants had a relaxed attitude towards six as a fixed target for their intake of fruits and vegetables, the number was still perceived as based on objective science and associated with a notion of self-discipline. Following the ideas of Espeland and Stevens, we can say that the campaign achieved a moral effect through the objective and scientific connotations of a precise number to convey the message: the numbers exerted a discipline on the targeted subjects (Espeland and Stevens (2008), p. 414), even though the target itself was not taken literally.

Our study showed that many of the informants shared a sense of scepticism towards the public health authorities and showed resistance to the connotations of 'control' associated with their way of communicating on health issues. The mould, '6 a day', however, was perceived as non-paternalistic, although still carrying a scientifically defined morality that was worth following. The hollow form of the mould appealed to the people's common sense and inclinations for freedom of choice, building on the assumption that individual skills in organizing and designing health practices could be relied upon. Since the number was not perceived as a target to be taken literally, almost anything that the citizens perceived as healthy could fit the mould. That the number in itself did not matter made it flexible, giving it the potential to contain heterogeneous sets of meanings to be tied to the micro management of the citizens' health practices.

How numbers influence everyday health practices

The number six from the campaign invited citizens to trust numbers, and also to multiply and produce numbers to design their own health practices. This said, some interviewees were relaxed and distanced in their attitudes towards numbers in health while others were more concerned with counting practices, adding to our insights about how numbers influence everyday health practices, and what kinds of practices are strengthened by moulds such as '6 a day'. Our interviews showed that when these informants managed to stick to numbers (of many kinds), it brought a sense of achievement and well-being. Using numbers as an organizing principle, healthy living came to the fore as a central motif, associated with a morality that stressed individual responsibility and self-regulation.

The cases of Poul and Anne Lise serve to illustrate and further explore this point. Both approached numbers as solid entities to be used as organizing principles in living a healthy life. Poul, aged 53, did not like the campaign '6 a day' at all, finding it rather silly, but nevertheless shared his concerns and preoccupations with his dietary regimen. This included eating 600 grams of what he called 'greens' as a daily target, achieved by making a smoothie each morning consisting principally of vegetables and fruits; he and his wife peeled and diced all the fruits and vegetables and put them into boxes on Sundays. When he shopped, he made use of 'the point diet' as a regimen and carefully checked and calculated the number of calories in each food item, with a daily calorie target in mind.

Anne Lise was a 67-year-old woman who suffered from diabetes and obesity. She had consulted a dietician who also advised her to establish a target for daily caloric intake. She aimed for a fixed number of 360 calories per main meal and 120 for snacks. In order to ease the burden of daily calculation, the dietician had provided her with a scheme listing all the food items she should eat with their exact number of calories. Moreover, the dietician had given her a shopping guide which provided her with exact figures for the amount of fat and fibre in different food categories (bread, dairy products, etc.). She combined this with other details, some of them originally from the '6 a day' campaign, for instance, that one decilitre of juice can substitute for one piece of fruit. Thus, the '6 a day' rule had become part of her personal repertoire of dietary guidelines, alongside other bodies of expert knowledge. Numbers in this case were made 'thick' (Geertz, 1973) by adding other numbers and layers of meanings, and by connecting them to different aspects of everyday life, such as dietary advice, supplementary knowledge, and cost calculations. For Anne Lise, as for many others, personal knowledge and dietary strategies served to link together practices such as the acts of buying and eating. Numbers became concrete, embodied entities and the means to develop a personal strategy.

Another example of this is Ditte, a 42-year-old secretary, who also used the numerical logic inherent in the mould '6 a day' but translated it even further to fit her personal knowledge and rules of thumb that reflected the logic of numbers. She had recently finished a course in nutrition and dreamed of becoming a nutritional consultant. Ditte did not recall other details from the campaign '6 a day', apart from the number and an unspecified recollection that it was 'quite old'. The notion of healthy self-management by numbers, however, was crucial for her everyday consumption practices. During the interview it emerged that, although she was eager to become an expert in nutrition and was very concerned about her own health, her awareness of, and interest in, public health information was very limited. She claimed to love measuring and quantifying; for instance, she carefully counted the calories and fat in each meal, she tracked her average speed every time she was jogging, and she used an app to watch her weight by the means of a graph. But Ditte was far from satisfied with the campaign '6 a day' as she found it too simplistic. In her view the number provided was insufficient. It needed to be integrated with a much more developed package of knowledge. As she said:

> I think that vegetables should fill more than half of my plate. I also eat fruit but it contains so much fructose that you should not eat six pieces a day; you should have a maximum of two and the rest vegetables.

Hence the numerical logic of the campaign mirrored her daily practices; she also used a calculative mould, although she filled it with her own material.

Using and fleshing out the mould from the campaign, numbers became personal for most of the informants, developing into an organizing principle for the arrangement of their everyday health practices. This empirical evidence supports Miller's (2004) point that practices of counting and quantifying may shape and transform human organization. The informants in the current study differ in their perceptions and practices, however. The above cases show that people may adopt the numerical logic of the mould to varying degrees, meaning that it can be seen as exerting a disciplinary power that reaches far beyond its actual message, even if the actual message is not taken very literally. Furthermore, most of the informants also used the numerical logic of the campaign's mould to externalize and communicate something about their personal identities. This was most salient in Ditte's case, as she integrated numbers and calculating practices into her narratives of who she was and wanted to be in the future; yet Bente also augmented her perception of being a woman with understandings from the campaign.

Discussion and conclusion

Numbers are appealing to the authorities as well as to citizens, as they communicate, offer perceptions of, and form health practices. This has been shown in former research and is confirmed by this study. The contribution of this article has been to provide a deeper understanding of how numbers in health campaigns may be appealing for the authorities and citizens, who both use numbers to navigate between simplicity and complexity, if in different yet reconcilable ways. Both take a pragmatic stance towards the numbers, but for divergent reasons; both value numbers for their simple, objective, and legitimate connotations, meanwhile filling out the spaces left by their inherent ambiguities dissimilarly. Citizens, on the other hand, add another layer of meaning, also using numbers to communicate about their personal identities.

Hence, numbers in health communications may be highly effective. However, the translations from the views of the authorities to those of citizens must be taken into consideration when we evaluate the actual impacts. The evaluation of health campaigns has for decades been closely related to health literacy. In order to regulate personal health, it is presumed that people can read and comprehend health messages, and take a position on these messages (Chinn, 2011; Nutbeam, 2008; Papen, 2009). This study has shown that people may take quite a different position on the message '6 a day' than might be expected if thinking along the lines of traditional health communications and health literacy. This was shown through analysis of the translations taking place as the '6 a day' catchphrase was created, disseminated, and taken up by citizens.

The different actors originally involved in designing the campaign (public authorities and private companies) negotiated and formed the mould, '6 a day', based on a combination of scientific and pragmatic rationales. Subsequently, in the translation process, certain elements of knowledge and understanding from the original campaign were preserved while others were adjusted. Ultimately, via this translation, the campaign constructed certain truths about health, and practices connected with health maintenance among Danish citizens (Latour, 1999, p. 24). Even though the mould was originally grounded in scientific evidence, ultimately pragmatic reasoning came to dominate the construction process. This demonstrates that the number used in the campaign, despite standing as a neutral scientific entity, is in fact a historical construct affected by different logics – in this case a scientific logic and a pragmatic logic which was more concerned with the communicative effects of the message and an awareness of international health trends and campaigns. These logics matter in the further translation processes of the campaign. In this case, a private company chose to produce a poster exploiting the sexual implications of the number six, thereby strengthening the pragmatic logic. However, the basic structure and scientific numerical logic of the mould were preserved, and our analysis showed that this structure was decisive for the perception of the campaign, as well as for the campaign's effect on informants' daily practice and their own communications about their identity.

Although people apparently did not pay much attention to the fixed number as such, they were nevertheless influenced by the implicit numerical logic with its connotations of absolutism and legitimacy. They assimilated the moral message 'to eat more fruit and vegetables' in their daily lives and perceived '6 a day' as a rule of thumb. They furthermore embraced the numerical logic as a valid way to design their own general health practices. While the number that was intended to form the contours of the mould appeared to be simple, objective and unquestionable, how people chose to fill the mould was far more varied. Being provided a hollow mould to fill with personal health knowledge and practices enabled substantial creativity and many different approaches to health among recipients. Common to those approaches which are shaped by the mould, however, are an inherent logic of numbers, the use of rule of thumb, and self-discipline and self-reliance as basic principles.

The campaign '6 a day' was disseminated as part of a 'pragmatic' strategy for improving public health. If measured in terms of its visibility and the familiarity of its logo, the campaign was highly successful. If the goal had been to improve health literacy among Danish citizens, the campaign does not seem to have attained it, as the number six has not added much to existing knowledge. This indicates that a focus on health literacy in public health campaigns as a criterion for success might miss the point. A campaign cannot be evaluated solely on whether the target audience actually understood and acted upon the concrete message. Instead, the implicit logic as well as the actual form of the campaign should be analysed, specifically its pragmatic purpose. We argue that future research could benefit from analysing the different logics that are involved in specific health campaigns, and how they influence the construction of the health message as well as perceptions among the targeted receivers of the message. As a concluding point, we therefore encourage stakeholders and scholars to pay greater attention to the underlying implications of a campaign and the effects and side effects of using moulds in health communications.

Notes

1. For instance, in a market analysis conducted between 2009 and 2011, 90% of Danes recognized that they had seen the campaign in the media. According to an estimate towards the beginning of the campaign the consumption of fruits and vegetables increased; however, after some years sales stagnated and have not increased in recent years. Moreover, the level of motivation to serve more vegetables and fruits dropped from 50 to 40% in the period 2009–2011 (Tranberg, 2011 internal report).
2. Landbrug og Fødevarer.

Acknowledgements

We want to thank Annemarie Mol and her group 'Eating Bodies' at the Department of Anthropology at the University of Amsterdam for their feedback on a very early draft. We also owe thanks to Morten Meyer Strunge, Thomas Derek Robinson, Domen Bajde, Nanna Ahlmark, Niklas Woermann, and Jessica Chelekis for their comments on the article.

Disclosure statement

No potential conflict of interest was reported by the authors.

Funding

This work was supported by the Helsefonden.

References

Anker, T., Kristensen, D., Brennan, L. (2015). Truth in social marketing. Social marketing Conference, Staffordshire, UK. In *Proceedings of the world social marketing conference (WSMC 2015)* (pp. 24–26). Staffordshire.

Callon, M. (2007). Some elements of a sociology of translation: Domestication of the scallops and the fishermen of St. Brieuc Bay. In K. Asdal, B. Brenna, & I. Moser (Eds.), *Technoscience. The politics of interventions* (pp. 57–79). Oslo: Oslo University Press.

Chinn, D. (2011). Critical health literacy: A review and critical analysis. *Social Science & Medicine, 73*, 60–67. doi:10.1016/j.socscimed.2011.04.004

Espeland, W. N., & Stevens, M. L. (2008). A sociology of quantification. *Archives Européennes de Sociologie* [European Journal of Sociology], *49*, 401–436. Retrieved from https://www.cambridge.org/core/journals/european-journal-of-sociology-archiveseuropeennes-de-sociologie

Geertz, C. (1973). *The interpretation of cultures.* New York, NY: Basic.

Kusenbach, M. (2003). Street phenomenology: The go-along as ethnographic research tool. *Ethnography, 4*, 455–485. doi:10.1177/146613810343007

Latour, B. (1991). Technology is society made durable. In J. Law (Ed.), *A sociology of monsters: Essays on power, technology and domination* (pp. 103–131). London: Routledge. (Sociological review monograph: 38).

Latour, B. (1999). *Pandora's hope. Essays on the reality of science studies.* Cambridge, MA: Harvard University Press.

Law, J. (2004). *After method. Mess in social science research.* New York, NY: Routledge.

Lomborg, S., & Frandsen, K. (2015). Self-tracking as communication. *Information, Communication and Society, 19*, 1015–1027. doi:10.1080/1369118X.2015.1067710

Lupton, D. (2013). Quantifying the body: Monitoring and measuring health in the age of mHealth technologies. *Critical Public Health, 23*, 393–403. doi:10.1057/sth.2013.10

Miles, B. M., Huberman, A. M., & Saldaña, J. (2014). *Qualitative data analysis – A methods sourcebook* (3rd ed.). Thousand Oaks, CA: Sage.

Miller, P. (2004). Governing by numbers. Why calculative practices matter. Chapter 10. In A. Amin & N. Trift (Eds.), *Cultural economy reader* (pp. 179–189). Oxford: Blackwell Publishing.

Mol, A. (2002). *The body multiple.* Durham and London: Duke University Press.

Nafus, D., & Sherman, J. (2014). This one does not go up to 11: The quantified self movement as an alternative bid data practice. *International Journal of Communication, 8*, 1784–1794. Retrieved from https://ijoc.org

Nutbeam, C. (2008). The evolving concept of health literacy. *Social Science & Medicine, 67*, 2072–2078.

Oxlund, B. (2012). Living by numbers: The dynamic interplay of asymptomatic conditions and low cost measurement technologies in the cases of two women in the Danish provinces. *Suomen Antropologi: The Journal of Finnish Anthropological Society, 37*, 42–56. Retrieved from https://journal.fi/suomenantropologi

Pantzer, M., & Ruckenstein, M. (2015). The heart of everyday analytics: Emotional, material and practical extensions in self tracking market. *Consumption, Market & Culture, 18*(1), 92–109. doi:10.1080/10253866.2014.899213

Papen, U. (2009). Literacy, learning and health – A social practices view of health literacy. *Literacy and Numeracy Studies, 16*, 19–34. doi:10.5130/lns.v0i0.1275

Poovey, M. (1998). *A history of the modern fact.* Chicago, IL: University of Chicago Press.

Porter, T. (1995). *Trust in numbers. The pursuit of objectivity in science and public life.* Princeton, NJ: Princeton University Press.

Sharon, T., & Zandbergen, D. (2016). From data fetishism to quantifying selves. Self-tracking practices and the other values of data. *New Media & Society.* doi:10.1177/1461444816636090

Timmerman, S., & Epstein, S. (2010). A world of standards but not a standard world: Toward a sociology of standards and standardization. *Annual Review of Sociology, 36*, 69–89. doi:10.1146/annurev.soc.012809.102629

Tranberg. (2011). *Tranberg market analysis.* Unpublished report.

Trolle, E., Fagt, S., & Ovesen, L. (1998). *Fruit and vegetables – Recommendations for intake.* Copenhagen: Ministry of Food, Agriculture and Fisheries of Denmark.

9 Newspaper coverage of childhood immunisation in Australia

A lens into conflicts within public health

Niamh Stephenson 🆔, Shefali Chaukra, Ilan Katz and Anita Heywood

ABSTRACT

Public health efforts to lift childhood vaccination rates can be supported or undermined by media representations of parents. Polarising representations neglect the large range of 'middle-ground' positions people occupy, potentially alienating parents. In recent years, Australian public health actors have tried to better engage journalists to avoid this. As these efforts have unfolded, the main national immunisation policy lever has become more punitive. This paper examines whether Australian newspaper representations of parents have changed, by comparing 153 newspaper articles from two periods: 1997–1998 (prior to the development of a public health lobby targeting the media; when the first national childhood immunisation policy was introduced) and; 2015–2016 (5 years after advocacy groups began working with the media; and when the national policy took a punitive turn). We analyse patterns and shifts (between 1997–1998 and 2015–2016) in the portrayal of parents as complacent, alternative, hesitant and as choosing. Australian newspaper portrayals of parents are broadly aligned with the policy targets of the day. In 2015–2016, there was less negative representation of parents who occupy the 'middle-ground' between vaccine acceptance and rejection. However, coverage of alternative parents (vaccine objectors) intensified in quantity and negativity. Concurrently, there were new (minority) portrayals of vaccine objectors as invisible, and as victims being denied choice. This signals that reporting may simultaneously align with national policy targets *and* destabilise public health efforts to avoid polarising misrepresentations of parents, characterisations likely to undermine trust in public health. Rather than 'blame the media', this analysis illuminates conflicts *within* public health.

The role of the media in shaping public engagement with childhood immunisation is of great interest to public health; reporting is understood to support or undermine public health objectives (Bubela et al., 2009; Downs, de Bruin, & Fischhoff, 2008; Keane et al., 2005). This is highlighted by enduring public fears about links between the Measles, Mumps, Rubella (MMR) vaccine and autism following the publicity surrounding Andrew Wakefield's study, which the UK General Medical Council deemed to be fraudulent. Media reporting of the MMR controversy fuelled mistrust and declines in vaccination rates (Petts & Niemeyer, 2004). Australian public health immunisation experts have been pro-actively engaging with the media in recent years. These actors include the familiar Federal and State/Territory Departments of Health officials, clinicians, public health experts and researchers. Additionally, since

2009 advocacy groups have been involved, such as Stop the Australian Vaccination Network (AVN) (national, founded in 2009), Northern Rivers Vaccination Supporters (working in an area with low vaccine coverage, founded in 2013) and the national Immunisation Coalition (founded 2015).

These advocacy groups' strategies have included encouraging journalists to desist adopting an impartial position on immunisation and then presenting 'two sides' of a debate (coverage which typically takes the form of public health expert opinion presented alongside spokespeople with opposing views). This journalistic approach can polarise opinions and create perceptions of a 'false balance' in public discussions (Gamson & Modigliani, 1989; Jackson, 2011). Additionally, under the rubric of Stop the AVN, public health actors ran a successful campaign (2010) to remove the charity status of the Australian Vaccination Network (AVN) – a vaccine questioning organisation. This decreased the AVN's access to resources and media coverage. The campaign also forced the AVN's name change, to the Australian Vaccination Skeptics Network (Dunlop, 2012, 2013). Hence, in addition to informing journalists about the evidence underpinning the vaccination schedule, concerted efforts have been made to interrupt oppositional reporting. Such reporting can complicate parents' efforts to inform themselves about immunisation; and can problematically perpetuate the misunderstanding that parents and wider publics are either pro- or anti-vaccination.

Over the last two decades, research into parents' engagement with vaccination has demonstrated that polarising accounts of parents as either 'acceptors' or 'non-acceptors' explain the positions of a minority of parents only. There is a range of 'middle ground' positions that parents take and potentially move through in their vaccine decision-making. For instance, Dubé et al. (2013) suggest that between acceptors and rejecters there are a large number of 'vaccine hesitant' parents with concerns about vaccination; notably their actions may encompass non-, partial or even full immunisation. In their review of 112 studies, Leask et al. (2012) further differentiate unquestioning acceptors (30–40%), cautious acceptors (25–35%), hesitant parents (20–30%), late or selective vaccinators (2–27%) and refusers (<2%) from each other. Leask et al. derive these categories from engagement with international literature, whilst the percentages they ascribe are based on US studies. Beyond concerns about safety, parents' decisions may be shaped by complacency and an underestimation of risk (Dubé et al., 2013; Leask et al., 2012; Tickner, Leman, & Woodcock, 2006). Additionally, parents who are socio-economically disadvantaged or isolated may not vaccinate due to barriers to access, a lack of social support, competing pressures in a large family or time pressures (Leask & Chapman, 2002; Pearce, Marshall, Bedford, & Lynch, 2015). Efforts to 'correct' parents' erroneous understandings of vaccination can be counterproductive and result in solidifying intentions to avoid vaccination (Nyhan, Reifler, Richey, & Freed, 2014).

Together, this body of research emphasises that public health efforts to promote childhood immunisation need to prioritise trust building. Public health works on multiple fronts to build trust in vaccination, e.g. vaccine monitoring and safety, training health care professionals in skilled one-on-one communications, and engaging in and with the media to shape public understandings and to avoid alienating parents via misrepresentation. Australian public health advocates' engagement with the media is part of this effort.

The work of public health advocacy groups such as Stop the AVN and The Immunisation Coalition has been informed by research into Australian newspaper coverage of immunisation (Leask & Chapman, 2002). This research identified problematically oppositional characterisations of parents in 1993–1998 coverage: journalists commonly created a narrative story with a villain, parents who did not vaccinate (Leask & Chapman, 2002). Reporting of 'both sides' of the immunisation debate, discussed above, was identified as having the potential to misinform and act as negative publicity for vaccinations (Leask & Chapman, 1998). Such findings highlight the potential for media to undermine public health efforts to acknowledge the majority of parents with a range of middle ground positions on vaccination – hence the extensive public health advocacy work undertaken since 2009.

This paper focuses on Australian public health actors' efforts to depolarise media coverage of immunisation. We examine the representations of parents in Australian newspaper stories on childhood immunisation, comparing recent (2015–2016) reporting with that of late 1990s (1997–1998). Between these two time periods, Stop the AVN was founded and has continued to be active alongside advocacy groups formed in 2013 and 2015. However, we cannot consider changes in newspaper reporting independently of the policy domain of Australian childhood immunisation, which has shifted substantially since 1997. When examining changes in newspaper representations of parents, below, we see that the current mismatch between Australian public health policy and practice is playing out in media reporting of parents, with potentially problematic consequences for public engagement with immunisation. Rather than 'blame the media', our analysis illuminates conflicts *within* public health

Australian immunisation policies and institutions

1997 policy developments

Australia's first National Immunisation Program (NIP) was instituted in 1997, in an effort to lift vaccination rates: at that time 75% of infants aged 12 months were fully vaccinated (McIntyre et al., 2000) and 53% of children under 6 (Taylor, Gray, & Stanton, 2016), far below 95% coverage targets. The NIP is a nationally funded programme, delivered under the directive of the eight individual States and Territories; it also funds the National Centre for Immunisation Research and Surveillance (NCIRS). The *first national* immunisation policy was launched in 1997 and implemented in 1998. It included incentives (bonus payments) for parents, which functioned by linking immunisation records with family assistance payments and tax benefits (Child Care Benefit, Child Care Rebate and Family Tax Benefit Part A supplement). Initially, general practitioners (GP) were also incentivised to report to the national Australian Childhood Immunisation Register (ACIR) and to achieve high practice coverage. The details of parents' incentives changed as the family assistance and national immunisation policies were modified between 1998 and 2015, but the fundamental policy lever remained the same: eligibility to some (not all) family benefits became conditional on immunisation status.

Importantly, the ACIR was established in 1996, as part of the Immunise Australia programme. The register included all children under 7 enrolled with the population-wide Medicare system (Australia's Medicare is akin to the UK's National Health Service [NHS]). Practitioners record vaccines given and can extract individual and practice reports from the ACIR. National, State and local level immunisation coverage is reported regularly. Until 2016, the ACIR included the option for parents to formally register their conscientious objection and so remain eligible for federal family payments. Objection required more than 'abstention', parents needed to consult with a GP who needed to first discuss the benefits of vaccination before registering the child. Hence, the 1997 policy (and its subsequent modifications prior to 2015) prompted all who wanted to avail of federal family benefits to choose to act in some way. ACIR records of conscientious objection increased from 0.23% of all registered children in 1999 to 1.77% in 2014 (likely indicating enhanced surveillance of this group rather than real significant increases) (Department of Health, 2015).

Via incentives and the ACIR the 1998 policy targeted parents deemed complacent or hesitant, triggering action to either immunise or register their objection. Recorded vaccination rates increased and then plateaued around 2000, with 2015 figures indicating 92.3 and 92.6% of children were up to date at 12 months and 5 years of age (Department of Health, 2017).

2015 policy developments

Australia's national childhood immunisation policy has taken a significantly different, punitive turn. The new national policy – known as *No Jab No Pay* – was announced in 2015, it came into effect in 2016 and was further refined in 2017. *No Jab No Pay* removes the option to register vaccine objection on the ACIR; only medical exemption remains. From 2016 on, families of unvaccinated or partially vaccinated children are ineligible to receive payments and tax benefits of up to $AU 15k per annum (depending on means testing, number of children and childcare arrangements)[1]. The 2016 policy target has shifted from complacent and hesitant parents to those who object. Removing the possibility to register vaccine objection removes parental 'choice' for parents who cannot afford to forgo state family support. Early indications suggest that in the first 6 months of 2016, coverage of 12 month olds rose by 0.94%–93.2% (Leask & Danchin, 2017). Additionally, as part of these developments the ACIR was expanded to include vaccines at all ages in 2016 and renamed the Australian Immunisation Register (AIR) in 2017.

The name of the 2016 policy, *No Jab No Pay*, echoes a New South Wales (NSW) newspaper campaign launched in May 2013. The *Daily Telegraph's No Jab No Play* campaign aimed to get 'the federal government to close a loophole enabling parents to claim they are "conscientious objectors" to avoid the rule that only vaccinated children are eligible for the … childcare rebate' (5 May 2013, *The Sunday Telegraph*). (Its second stated aim was to have unvaccinated children banned from NSW childcare centres). Whilst the newspaper claimed the national policy change as their 'stunning victory' (11 April 2015, *Daily Telegraph*), the *No Jab No Pay* policy has triggered extensive controversy within the Australian public health community.

The rationale for punitively targeting vaccine objection has been debated within public health. This minority group of parents accounts for less than 20% of all children in Australia who are not fully immunised (Leask & Danchin, 2017; Wiley, Cooper, Wood, & Leask, 2015). Public health actors know that health inequalities and social determinants shape patterns of incomplete and non-vaccination, e.g. migration, social isolation, support, stress and social gradients (Attwell, Leask, Meyer, Rokkas, & Ward, 2017; Cashman et al., 2016; Pearce et al., 2015). Children who are not fully vaccinated, but have no recorded conscientious objection, are more likely than fully vaccinated children to be in the lowest socio-economic decile or overseas born (Beard, Hull, Leask, Dey, & McIntyre, 2016). The 2016 policy's negative impact on some already socially disadvantaged groups, such as migrant children and their families, could have been predicted (Paxton, Oldfield, Kiang, & Danchin, 2016). Concerns around choice-restricting approaches, such as *No Jab No Pay*, include that even if effective in raising coverage in the short term, punitive policies may alienate groups of parents whom public health actors have been striving to win over to vaccination (Kitta & Goldberg, 2017; Leask & Danchin, 2017) – including but also beyond those with strong objections.

Clearly, the timeframe during which public health actors have tried to engage the media (to avoid polarising characterisation of parents) is marked with a significant policy shift. This fluid policy terrain adds to the significance to our question about whether research about the importance of acknowledging parents' diverse approaches to immunisation is being reflected in media coverage of vaccination. The media's alignment with public health research and practice matters because reporting can play an important role in proliferating polarising representations of parents, of the kind that can alienate parents from health professionals and public health. Hence, this paper seeks to understand how parents are being characterised in Australian media about childhood immunisation. We do this by comparing Australian newspaper representations of parents' positions on vaccination during two timeframes; in 1997–1998 (before the formation of public health advocacy groups who have worked intensively with the media; the period of the introduction of the first national programme and policy and immunisation incentives); and 2015–2016 (after the formation of advocacy groups, the time when a strong punitive lever was added to national policy).

Methods

Data collection

We selected the highest circulating national newspaper (*The Australian*) and four metropolitan newspapers with the highest readerships (*The Age, Herald-Sun, Daily Telegraph, The Sydney Morning Herald,* and corresponding Sunday papers), using Ray Morgan data (a market research company, whose remit includes advertising research). We conducted two searches via the Factiva database for articles referring to parents and vaccination[2], restricting the size of the data-set by selecting the two time periods during which Australian childhood immunisation policy underwent the greatest changes. The first search (1 January 1997–31 December 1998) covered the announcements of the first NIP (1997) and the first national childhood immunisation policy in 1998 (discussed above). The second (1 March 2015–30 June

2016) covered the period of one month before the announcement of *No Jab No Pay* to 6 months after its implementation (i.e. covering the period during which punitive policy measures were introduced). The exact search terms were: (Vaccinate* OR vaccination* or vaccinating or immunise* or immunisation* or immunising or immunize* or immunization* or immunizing*) AND (child* or kid* or infant*) AND (parent* or mum or mums or dad* or mother* or father*). We identified 72 articles from the 1997 to 1998 search and 109 articles from the 2015 to 2016 search. Of these 8 articles from 1997 to 1998 and 20 from 2015 to 2016 were excluded because they were duplicates, irrelevant to childhood vaccination, or internationally focused. The final data-set comprised 153 articles; 64 from 1997 to 1998 and 89 from 2015 to 2016.

Thematic coding and analysis

The final data-set of 153 articles was uploaded into NVivo software for qualitative data coding and analysis. A descriptive coding schedule was developed, via examination of a subset of 20 articles (selected from a range of newspapers across both time periods) to identify the positions explicitly or implicitly assigned to parents. The coding schedule was developed with the broad research question in mind: how are parents being represented? Initially, codes were deductively derived from our analysis of existing research (e.g. 'disadvantaged', 'hesitant', 'complacent'). Additional, inductive codes were added to ensure inclusion of data relevant to our interest in the representation of parents (e.g. 'the crowd').

The schedule was then piloted on a further 20 articles, to ensure inter-coder reliability and to iteratively refine codes (some codes were merged). This resulted in nine codes (see Table 1), each capturing a distinct (although occasionally overlapping) representation of parents in news media. These nine codes were then used to code the complete data-set in NVivo. Where relevant, sections of articles were double-coded (e.g. if both parents were evoked as both hesitant and as choosers). In total, 635 sections were coded (267 in 1997–1998 data and 368 in 2015–2016). Thus, coding yielded a description of the data-set, in the form of patterns in the characterisation of parents, within and between time periods.

We present these patterns below, using quotes to illustrate, before focusing on select patterns as raising questions for further analysis (Scott, 1991; Stephenson & Papadopoulos, 2006). Specifically, we focus on shifts (between 1997–1998 and 2015–2016) in the portrayal of parents as complacent, alternative, hesitant and as choosing. These particular changes, as we discuss below, raise questions about the complex relationships between media representations and policy, practice and research regarding public health's engagement with or alienation of parents. They signal that media may simultaneously (a) align with public health research avoiding *some* oversimplified, polarising portrayals of parents, and (b) support public health policy with the intensification of problematically polarised media representations of parents. Our analysis, below, points to divergences between national immunisation policy and public health research on the most effective ways of engaging parents.

Table 1. Descriptive coding schedule of representations of parents.

Code	Description of code
Good parents	Parents who fully vaccinate; typically cast as role models who uphold the social norm
Hesitant parents	Unsure or concerned; sometimes portrayed as over-anxious, at other times normalised
Parents as choosers	Making or wanting choice; characterised positively (e.g. intelligent) or negatively (e.g. selfish)
Complacent parents	Ignorant, apathetic, negligent, lazy and/or forgetful
Alternative parents	Deliberately choose to not vaccinate their children because of moral or religious beliefs, lifestyle choices, or concerns about vaccine safety or effectiveness; sometimes characterised as 'crusaders', threats to society or irrational, at other times portrayed as victims
Irresponsible parents	Parents' lack of action implicitly or explicitly characterised as irresponsible
The crowd	Parents characterised *as a group* capable of being swayed either into becoming 'Good Parents' or by anti-vaccination lobbies to 'Alternatives'
Disadvantaged parents	Socio-economic disadvantage, access barriers
Medically exempt	Vaccination is contraindicated due to medical reasons

Findings

Australian newspaper coverage of parents often avoids over-simplistically representing parents as pro or anti-vaccination. Some of the more nuanced positions (e.g. hesitancy, complacency) that have been identified by public health researchers as contributing to patterns in vaccination are evident in newspaper reporting, in both 1997–1998 and 2015–2016 (see Figure 1).

Clearly however, correspondence between what is known about parents whose children are not fully vaccinated and newspaper representations is low. For instance, in both time periods only 4.1% of the coded data-sets raised social disadvantage or social determinants of health as pertinent to parents' actions, whilst research indicates that these factors are paramount for up to 80% of children who are not fully immunised (Attwell et al., 2017; Cashman et al., 2016; Pearce et al., 2015).

Notable shifts in frequency of some characterisations of parents are also evident, indicated in Figure 1. Representations of parents as complacent comprised 10.9% of the coded data-set in 1997–1998, but dropped to 6% in 2015–2016. Coverage of parents characterised as alternative increased considerably, from 10.1% of the coded data in 1997–1998 to 30.4% in 2015–2016. The portrayal of parents as 'choosers' decreased (from 10.9 to 5.7%). There was little change in the proportion of media coverage in which parents were characterised as hesitant (from 7.5 to 6.8%). Frequency changes aside, there were some shifts in the way particular parental positions were characterised, e.g. with more generous characterisations of hesitant and complacent parents in 2015–2016.

Below, we analyse these shifts in the levels and nature of media interest, specifically examining the forms of polarising newspaper coverage of parents that public health actors have been explicitly trying to interrupt.

Less polarising coverage of hesitant and complacent parents in 2015–2016 reporting

As discussed above, beyond designating parents as 'acceptors' or 'non-acceptors', public health researchers have identified groups of complacent, selective and hesitant parents. This research characterises hesitant parents as engaging with vaccination (although sometimes late) but having concerns around safety and risk. It proposes that acknowledging and addressing (rather than discounting) such concerns may result in full, timely immunisation (Leask et al., 2012).

Whilst the frequency of newspaper coverage of hesitant parents changed little over time, its nature altered considerably. In 1997–1998, hesitant parents were commonly negatively portrayed as

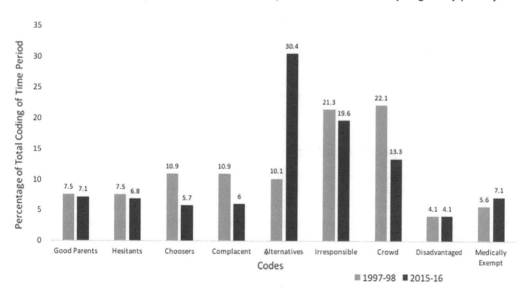

Figure 1. The percentage of each code in 1997–1998 and 2015–2016 data-sets.

over-anxious, recalcitrant or lacking the 'right' information or education (a notion that research does not substantiate). Consider for instance: '... their concerns about immunisation are unfounded since much of the anxiety about side-effects of vaccines is based on wrong or outdated information' (26 February 1997, *The Age*). In contrast, in 2015–2016, less disparagement of parents' hesitancy was evident, e.g.: 'Care should be taken not to hector or demonise hesitant parents because this is counterproductive' (17 April 2015, *The Australian*).

Moreover, in 2015–2016, newspaper coverage commonly explored the concerns of hesitant parents in relative depth, e.g.: 'Critics of vaccination ... [include] "reformists" who largely accept vaccination but are critical or wary of some aspects (vaccine hesitancy)' (28 August 2015, *Sydney Morning Herald*). Thus, in contemporary reporting it was more common to see parents' questions being normalised and a new legitimacy being conferred on parents' concerns. In some cases, hesitant parents' *potential* to become 'good parents' is explicitly invoked, e.g. '... some parents who are neutral may be persuaded to vaccinate their child' (12 June 2016, *Sun-Herald*). Moreover, there is some acknowledgement that the solution may lie in building trust rather than simple factual education, e.g.: '... [a] new tailored approach to dealing with parents who are hesitant to vaccinate their children ... relies on building their trust and being non-judgmental, rather than bombarding them with facts and figures' (1 March 2015, *Herald-Sun*). The 2015–2016 newspaper coverage of parents' hesitancy clearly makes *some* of the questions parents might have about immunisation more visible. Moreover, it suggests that a level of parental concern is being legitimised – as part of the pathway towards vaccination.

A similar normalisation was evident in the shift in newspaper accounts of complacency between 1997–1998 and 2015–2016. In 2015–2016, coverage of complacency decreased, mirroring changes in policy. (In 1998, the national policy prompted complacent parents to either vaccinate or formally register vaccine objection, to ensure access to family benefits; this emphasis later changed as *No Jab No Pay* targets 'objectors'). Newspaper reports in 1997–1998 identified complacency as a problem, for instance: 'Dr .Wooldridge's [the then Federal Health Minister] target is not the parents who actively oppose immunisation, but the far larger group who fail to complete their children's immunisation, through apathy ... or indifference' (26 February 1997, *The Age*). At times reporting was alarmist, e.g. 'a frightening level of complacency has developed' (27 February 1997 *The Age*) or 'complacency and ignorance has let child immunisation coverage be a shameful 53 per cent' (4 March 1997, *The Age*). Complacent parents were described as negligent, e.g. for 'not bothering [and] ... leaving [their children] vulnerable to potentially fatal diseases' (8 July 1998, *The Age*). Such negative characterisations can be read as affirming the policy target of the day: problematic complacency. In addition to garnering less media interest, in 2015–2016, complacent parents were portrayed more charitably, e.g. as having 'fallen behind on their child's vaccination schedule for a variety of reasons' (17 April 2016, *Daily Telegraph*), or as busy parents 'simply forget[ting]' (21 Dec 2015, *The Age*).

Seen together, the more generous reporting of hesitancy and complacency in 2015–2016 might indicate that newspaper coverage is not only broadly supportive of policy shifts, but is becoming more closely aligned with public health efforts to avoid unnecessarily polarising parents. However, the intensified interest in alternative parents in 2015–2016 complicates such conclusions.

More polarising coverage of alternative parents in 2015–2016

In 1997–1998, parents characterised as alternatives were largely treated as a small group of people invested in alternative lifestyle and health practices. Their beliefs and practices were commonly ridiculed, e.g.: 'Public health expert Professor Simon Chapman says groups against immunisation were using conspiracy theories to blame everything from autism to criminality on vaccinations' (4 November 1998, *Daily Telegraph*). There were also some explicit characterisations of this group as a threatening public menace, e.g.: 'These people ... may have influenced a sizeable chunk of the adult population to stay away from vaccine jabs' (4 March 1997, *The Age*). As illustrated here, the threat was commonly characterised as the potential for alternative parents to influence the decision-making of other parents trying to make informed decisions.

Alternative parents were not always portrayed as a threat in 1997–1998. Reports included accurate accounts of their relatively low numbers, and affirmations of parental choice, e.g.: '… only 2 per cent of parents have a strong conscientious objection … "People have the right to opt out but they don't have the right to do nothing," he said' (26 February 1997, *The Age*). The 1998 policy's respect of choice was frequently supported, e.g. '[the policy] makes democratic allowance for … parents who have serious conscientious objections' (27 February 1997, *The Age*). Thus, although the 1997–1998 coverage of alternative parents was largely negative, the role that they might play in the shaping the national vaccination rates was often described in terms of a specific threat, and their right to choose affirmed. This media attention to specificity and rights changes in 2015–2016.

The 2015–2016 coverage of alternative parents triples in frequency (see Figure 1). This shift tracks changes in federal immunisation policy (rather than real increases in numbers of alternative parents) as *No Jab No Pay* targets vaccine objectors. By eliminating the mechanism for vaccine objectors to access significant family benefits, the 2016 policy frames objection as socially unacceptable. Newspaper stories in 2015–2016 commonly echoed this, presenting a different picture of the 'problem' of alternatives to that in 1997–1998 coverage. There was more ridicule in 2015–2016, and more vilification of alternative positions, e.g.: 'anti-vax quacks [who] are a tough crowd to shift. If the pure science and indisputable disease statistics don't convince them then who knows what will' (17 January 2016, *Daily Telegraph*). On occasion, the chastisement was extreme, e.g.: 'Anti-vaxers have a special seat reserved for them at hell's dinner table, right next to Holocaust deniers and those who think 9/11 was an inside job' (28 January 2016, *Daily Telegraph*).

In one sense, this negativity is continuous with that already evident in 1997–1998 characterisations of the threat that non- or partial vaccination poses to the health of others (through lowering herd immunity or through disease transmission). 2015–2016 reporting amplifies representations of alternative parents as putting 'their communities … at risk' (9 January 2016, *Herald-Sun*); or as a 'dangerous army of parents' (22 November 2015, *Herald-Sun*); and as responsible for a supposed 'upsurge of deadly diseases' (28 June 2015, *Herald-Sun*).

In another sense, there were discontinuities between reporting of alternative parents in 1997–1998 and 2015–2016. Firstly, alterative parents were newly characterised as an invisible threat in 2015–2016. For instance:

> In their day-to-day dealings, their innocent but unvaccinated kids are mixing with ours. And we are none the wiser because a growing number of deluded vaccine haters are keeping their fanaticism a secret. …. And being a new, silent risk to us and our children is their greatest crime of all. (28th January 2016, *Daily Telegraph*)

New concerns about the supposed concealment of alternative parents may be connected to *No Jab No Pay*'s attempt to render vaccine objection socially unacceptable. Perhaps it is envisaged by some that this strong signal will result in less disclosure – and more invisibility – on the part of alternative parents. Another possibility is that this spectre of dangerously invisible alternate parents is an unintended consequence of disbanding the option of registering vaccine conscientious objection. The ACIR/AIR closed this segment of the register in 2016 on the grounds that the rationale for its creation – to enable vaccine objectors to differentiate themselves from complacent parents by registering their stance and so continue to access State family benefits – had disappeared with the introduction of *No Jab No Pay*. In addition to the obviously problematical epidemiological gap this change leaves, our analysis suggests that the change may *also* be contributing to newspaper representations of the now 'secret' problem of alternative parents.

A second shift in coverage of alternative parents was apparent in reporting of parental 'choice'.

Increasingly polarised 2015–2016 reporting of parental choice reflects policy shifts

Australian childhood immunisation policy has shifted from promoting (1998) to removing (2016) choice. In 1998, childhood immunisation policy allowed parents to choose between immunisation and registering as a conscientious objector to vaccination, aiming to reduce complacency and hesitancy. Although the 1997–1998 reporting included a few accounts that problematised parental choice, like policy at that time, it largely affirmed parental choice about vaccination (e.g. as 'democratic'), e.g.: 'Dr. Wooldridge [the then Federal Health Minister] stands firm: "We are not promoting compulsory vaccination but rather compulsory effort"' (26 February 1997, *The Age*).

With the removal of choice via *No Jab No Pay*, in 2015–2016, coverage of parents as choosers dropped to 5.7%, from 10.9% in 1997–1998. Moreover, choice was increasingly portrayed as selfish, with comments such as 'placing freedom of choice above community welfare' (18 February 2016, *The Age*). The 2016 policy's limiting of parental choice was commonly supported, e.g. as 'saving young lives [and] protecting parents from themselves' (14 February 2016, *Daily Telegraph*). Support was not restricted to the campaigning Telegraph, for instance this national broadsheet reported:

> The policy does something important … it reinforces the idea vaccination is a social practice. The previous policy said 'vaccination is good but we don't mind if you don't do it'. The new policy says 'vaccination is good, and not doing it comes with a cost'. (17th April 2015, *The Australian*)

Hence, the second shift in coverage of alternative parents was, in 2015–2016, their choices were increasingly cast as a form of negligence that threatens 'our' children.

Before further considering this connection between reporting and policy approaches to alternative parents, we want to note the third shift in characterisations of such parents. A new, minority, representation was evident in 2015–2016, one which arguably cuts across the increased polarisation in representations of alternative parents – as victims being denied choice. Reporting included claims that 'the policy was unfair' (1 March 2015, *Herald-Sun*) and discussions of parents' rights. Traces of a (minority) notion of anti-vaccination as a 'pro-choice' stance were already evident in 1997–1998. However, in 2015–2016 it was more commonly affirmed, e.g. 'I am not against vaccinations; I am for pro-choice for everyone. We need the right to choose' (5 July 2015, *Daily Telegraph*). Thus, support for a policy that limits individual choice for the sake of collective health interests was not uniformly invoked in newspaper coverage.

Australian public health actors have worked extensively to move beyond polarising approaches to parents both in their own practices and in media representations. The 2015–2016 newspaper reporting of hesitancy and complacency might indicate some success: these positions are discussed in more generous and potentially less alienating terms. However, when we consider the intensified disparagement of alternative parents in 2015–2016 reporting, it seems that the imperative to avoid unnecessary polarisation has not been appropriated. Perhaps the villain role has shifted in line with policy targets. Some might invoke a ready at hand explanation: i.e. to 'blame the media' for reframing rather than moving beyond stories that hinge on a villain. However, this does not explain our finding that newspaper reporting can simultaneously align with *policy* shifts (i.e. intensified interest in and negativity towards alternatives) and diverge from *public health research and practice* objectives (to avoid alienating the target audience with polarising representations).

Discussion and conclusions

Public health efforts to work with the media still face considerable challenges. Firstly, the sheer growth of denigrating newspaper portrayals of alternative parents between 1997–1998 and 2015–2016 suggests an ongoing need to address adversarial reporting. Even in the form of advocacy, adversarial reporting can perpetuate *more* coverage of the views of a small minority of parents and increase polarisation (Leask, 2015). Whilst it is likely intended to affirm a policy designed to shift social norms, the increased vilification of alternative parents may work *against* public health efforts to lift vaccination rates by building trust.

Secondly, we have identified some new characterisations of alterative parents emerging in 2015–2016 reporting. One pertains to their supposed secretiveness and invisibility. This new representation of the 'threat' alternative parents may align with *No Jab No Pay*'s objective to render non-vaccination socially unacceptable. This problematic mode of polarising parents may also be an unintended consequence of the 2016 closure of the register of conscientious objectors.

Thirdly, whilst representations of parents as choosers decreased in 2015–2016, in step with the policy shift, they also changed in nature. Portrayals of choice largely shifted from a democratic right to deniable for the sake of the common good – but not entirely. *No Jab No Pay*'s 'fairness' was also questioned with representations of alternative parents as victims. Will such reframing of anti-vaccination and middle ground positions as pro-choice fuel concerns about parental rights and policy equity and fairness? If *No Jab No Pay* proves to have a sustained impact on vaccination coverage, this contestation of lack of choice signals that we will still need to ask if increases in vaccination rates reflect changes in social norms or a divergence between immunisation practices and social norms. As Geelen, van Vliet, de Hoogh, and Horstman (2016) demonstrate, when high vaccination rates are achieved at the expense of parents' negotiation and choice we cannot presume that they equate with trust in public health. Our findings indicate the potential for a new challenge for public health actors striving to gain public trust: newspaper coverage that extends the notion that anti-vaccination is essentially pro-choice may legitimise the anti-vaccination and middle ground positions that *No Jab No Pay* aims to undermine. A policy move understood by the public as limiting choice may *add* to the challenges already entailed in lifting vaccination rates (i.e. challenges to facilitate access, to communicate the rationale for the programme and to communicate facts about vaccine safety and effectiveness) (Macintyre & Salmon, 2015). Beyond childhood immunisation, public concerns about the denial of choice may affect trust in the institution of public health more broadly.

Clearly, our findings suggest that the Australian NIP does not entail a singular, unitary approach that can be traced through research, practice and policy. Rather, childhood immunisation is better understood as a network, or apparatus, of disparate discourses, institutions, entities and events which coalesce around a common object (Collier, Lakoff, & Rabinow, 2004; Foucault, 1994; Ong & Collier, 2005; Papadopoulos, Stephenson, & Tsianos, 2008) – in this case lifting childhood immunisation coverage. This foregrounds that immunisation policies, public health practices and research can converge, but also diverge. Our analysis points towards a divergence between (a) public health practitioners and advocates who – because they prioritise the importance of recognising the range of positions parents might navigate as they consider immunisation – are working to disrupt the polarisation of parents, and (b) a punitive policy which disregards these concerns. From this perspective, we can conclude that shifts in newspaper reporting of parents' positions on immunisation suggest something beyond journalists' partial appropriation of public health research on the large 'middle ground' of parents. Shifts in media reporting illustrate important divergences within Australian public health – between efforts to avoid polarisation, and a recent policy change that unleashes it. Following Paul, Wallenburg, and Bal (2018), we can see this as a case of 'infrastructural frictions' – frictions between the techniques used by policy-makers and public health practitioners to frame and address parents of unvaccinated or partially vaccinated children, all working under the NIP.

Moreover, it would be a mistake to presume that shifts in reporting follow on from policy changes. Increased negative reporting about alternative parents in 2015–2016 *may* be legitimised by, or even result from, media support for changes to immunisation policy. However, the media is part of, not outside of, the apparatus of childhood immunisation. Disparaging reporting can be seen as a technique used in a growing media campaign (The Telegraph's, discussed above) to shape policy. Approaching childhood immunisation as an apparatus which *includes* the media complicates the common sense delineation between 'public health' and 'media'; it also indicates the need for *specific* interrogation of the points of connection being formed, tested and reworked around childhood immunisation. Thus, the implications of this analysis are not simply that public health advocates need to renew their efforts to communicate with journalists and shape media coverage of childhood immunisation. It points towards the risk of blaming the media for what might be 'pragmatic amplification' of lines being fed by public health actors (Nerlich & Halliday, 2007, p. 62). Equally, it signals the risk of conflating media support for a policy, which discharges and directs negativity towards parents cast as alternatives, with support for public health practice and advocacy that strives to move beyond such polarisation.

Notes

1. State support for Australian families is in the form of welfare payments called 'tax benefits A and B' (rather than tax credits or tax breaks which alter regular take-home pay). In 2013, about 2/3rds of Australian children were being raised in families receiving tax benefits A and/or B. Of these, 35% received the full amount and 18% received the 'base rate' (around 1.6k) of Family Tax A (the larger of the 2 benefits) with the remainder on sliding scale between, dependant on family income (Whiteford & Crosby, 2015).
2. The Factiva database has the most comprehensive coverage of Australian newspaper archives from 1997 to 2016. However, it only includes the Sunday or weekend editions of three of the five newspapers selected (not for *The Sydney Morning Herald/ The Sun-Herald* and *The Age/Sunday Age*). Thus, two additional searches were conducted with the Proquest database to capture 1997–1998 and 2015–2016 coverage in *The Sun-Herald* and *Sunday Age*.

Disclosure statement

No potential conflict of interest was reported by the authors.

ORCID

Niamh Stephenson (iD) http://orcid.org/0000-0001-8105-1931

References

Attwell, K., Leask, J., Meyer, S., Rokkas, P., & Ward, P. (2017). Vaccine rejecting parents' engagement with expert systems that inform vaccination programs. *Journal of Bioethical Inquiry, 14*(1), 65–76. doi:10.1007/s11673-016-9756-7

Beard, F., Hull, B., Leask, J., Dey, A., & McIntyre, P. (2016). Trends and patterns in vaccination objection, Australia, 2002–2013. *The Medical Journal of Australia, 204*(7), 275.

Bubela, T., Nisbet, M., Borchelt, R., Brunger, F., Critchley, C., Einsiedel, E., ... Caufield, T. (2009). Science communication reconsidered. *Nature Biotechnology, 27*(6), 514–518.

Cashman, P. M., Allan, N. A., Clark, K. K., Butler, M. T., Massey, P. D., & Durrheim, D. N. (2016). Closing the gap in Australian Aboriginal infant immunisation rates – The development and review of a pre-call strategy. *BMC Public Health, 16*(1), 514. doi:10.1186/s12889-016-3086-x

Collier, S., Lakoff, A., & Rabinow, P. (2004). Biosecurity: Towards an anthropology of the contemporary. *Anthropology Today, 20*(5), 3–7.

Department of Health. (2015). ACIR – National vaccine objection (Conscientious objection) data'. Retrieved August 3, 2017, from http://www.immunise.health.gov.au/internet/immunise/publishing.nsf/Content/acir-cons-object-hist.htm

Department of Health. (2017). AIR – Annual coverage historical data. Retrieved August 3, 2017, from http://www.immunise.health.gov.au/internet/immunise/publishing.nsf/Content/acir-ann-cov-hist-data.htm

Downs, J., de Bruin, W., & Fischhoff, B. (2008). Parents' vaccination comprehension and decisions. *Vaccine, 26*(12), 1595–1607. doi:10.1016/j.vaccine.2008.01.011

Dubé, E., Laberge, C., Guay, M., Bramadat, P., Roy, R., & Bettinger, J. (2013). Vaccine hesitancy: An overview. *Human Vaccines & Immunotherapeutics, 9*(8), 1763–1773.

Dunlop, R. (2012). Anti-vaccination network told to change its name or be shut down. Retrieved August 3, 2017, from https://theconversation.com/anti-vaccination-network-told-to-change-its-name-or-be-shut-down-11368

Dunlop, R. (2013, October 16). Anti-vaccination activists should not be given a say in the media. *The Guardian*. Retrieved August 3, 2017, from https://www.theguardian.com/commentisfree/2013/oct/16/anti-vaccination-activists-should-not-be-given-a-say-in-the-media

Foucault, M. (1994). *Dits et écrits: Tome III, 1976–1979*. Paris: Gallimard.

Gamson, W., & Modigliani, A. (1989). Media discourse and public opinion on nuclear power: A constructionist approach. *American Journal of Sociology, 95*(1), 1–37.

Geelen, E., van Vliet, H., de Hoogh, P., & Horstman, K. (2016). Taming the fear of voice: Dilemmas in maintaining a high vaccination rate in the Netherlands. *Social Science & Medicine, 153*(Supplement C), 12–19.

Jackson, T. (2011). When balance is bias. *BMJ, 343*, d8006. doi:10.1136/bmj.d8006

Keane, M. T., Walter, M. V., Patel, B. I., Moorthy, S., Stevens, R. B., Bradley, K. M., ... Vernon, T. M. (2005). Confidence in vaccination: A parent model. *Vaccine, 23*(19), 2486–2493. doi:10.1016/j.vaccine.2004.10.026

Kitta, A., & Goldberg, D. S. (2017). The significance of folklore for vaccine policy: Discarding the deficit model. *Critical Public Health, 27*(4), 506–514. doi:10.1080/09581596.2016.1235259

Leask, J. (2015). Should we battle antivaccinationists? *Public Health Research & Practice, 25*(2), 1–4. doi:10.17061/phrp2521515

Leask, J., & Chapman, S. (1998). 'An attempt to swindle nature': Press anti-immunisation reportage 1993–1997. *Australian and New Zealand Journal of Public Health, 22*(1), 17–26. doi:10.1111/j.1467-842X.1998.tb01140.x

Leask, J., & Chapman, S. (2002). 'The cold hard facts' immunisation and vaccine preventable diseases in Australia's newsprint media 1993–1998. *Social Science and Medicine, 54*(3), 445–457.

Leask, J., & Danchin, M. (2017). Imposing penalties for vaccine rejection requires strong scrutiny. *Journal of Paediatrics and Child Health, 53*(5), 439–444.

Leask, J., Kinnersley, P., Jackson, C., Cheater, F., Bedford, H., & Rowles, G. (2012). Communicating with parents about vaccination: A framework for health professionals. *BMC Pediatrics, 12*, 154.

Macintyre, R., & Salmon, D. (2015, April 15). Want to boost vaccination? Don't punish parents, build their trust. *The Conversation*. Retrieved August 3, 2017, from https://theconversation.com/want-to-boost-vaccination-dont-punish-parents-build-their-trust-40094

McIntyre, P., Amin, J., Gidding, H., Hull, H., Torvaldsen, B., Tucker, A., … Burgess, M. (2000). *Vaccine preventable diseases and vaccination coverage in Australia, 1993–8*. Canberra: Union Offset: Communicale Diseases Network Australia.

Nerlich, B., & Halliday, C. (2007). Avian flu: The creation of expectations in the interplay between science and the media. *Sociology of Health & Illness, 29*(1), 46–65. doi:10.1111/j.1467-9566.2007.00517.x

Nyhan, B., Reifler, J., Richey, S., & Freed, G. L. (2014). Effective messages in vaccine promotion: a randomized trial. *Pediatrics, 133*, e835–e842. doi:10.1542/peds.2013-2365

Ong, A., & Collier, S. (2005). *Global assemblages : Technology, politics, and ethics as anthropological problems*. Malden, MA: Blackwell Publishing.

Papadopoulos, D., Stephenson, N., & Tsianos, V. (2008). *Escape routes: Power and control in the 21st century*. London: Pluto.

Paul, K. T., Wallenburg, I., & Bal, R. (2018). Putting public health infrastructures to the test: Introducing HPV vaccination in Austria and the Netherlands. *Sociology of Health & Illness, 40*(1), 67–81. doi:10.1111/1467-9566.12595

Paxton, G., Oldfield, S., Kiang, K., & Danchin, M. (2016). No Jab, No Pay – No planning for migrant children. *The Medical Journal of Australia, 205*(7), 296–298.

Pearce, A., Marshall, H., Bedford, H., & Lynch, J. (2015). Barriers to childhood immunisation: Findings from the longitudinal study of Australian children. *Vaccine, 33*(29), 3377–3383. doi:10.1016/j.vaccine.2015.04.089

Petts, J., & Niemeyer, S. (2004). Health risk communication and amplification: Learning from the MMR vaccination controversy. *Health, Risk & Society, 6*(1), 7–23. doi:10.1080/13698570410001678284

Scott, J. W. (1991). The evidence of experience. *Critical Inquiry, 17*(4), 773–797.

Stephenson, N., & Papadopoulos, D. (2006). *Analysing everyday experience. Social research and political change*. London: Palgrave Macmillan.

Taylor, D. R., Gray, M., & Stanton, D. (2016). New conditionality in Australian social security policy. *Australian Journal of Social Issues, 51*(1), 3–26. doi:10.1002/j.1839-4655.2016.tb00362.x

Tickner, S., Leman, P. J., & Woodcock, A. (2006). Factors underlying suboptimal childhood immunisation. *Vaccine, 24*(49–50), 7030–7036. doi:10.1016/j.vaccine.2006.06.060

Whiteford, P., & Crosby, M. (2015, May 11). FactCheck: Is half to two-thirds of the Australian population receiving a government benefit? *The Conversation*. Retrieved August 3, 2017, from https://theconversation.com/factcheck-is-half-to-two-thirds-of-the-australian-population-receiving-a-government-benefit-41027

Wiley, K., Cooper, S., Wood, N., & Leask, J. (2015). Understanding pregnant women's attitudes and behavior toward influenza and pertussis vaccination. *Qualitative Health Research, 25*(3), 360–370. doi:10.1177/1049732314551061

10 Is social isolation a public health issue?

A media analysis in Aotearoa/New Zealand

Mary Breheny (iD) and Christina Severinsen

ABSTRACT

Recognition of the health effects of social isolation has led to the media framing it as a public health issue. In this paper, we examine how the media frame social isolation among older people and how the public respond to this framing. Using framing analysis, we analysed an online article, embedded video content and 369 comments posted in response to this article. The article used a recognisable public health framing to understand the causes of social isolation as structural, supported by a video which presented the private face of a public health problem. The online comments largely resisted this framing, arguing that social isolation reflected an individual deficit, best remedied through individual actions such as joining groups or having a positive attitude. Families were also viewed as responsible for the social lives of their members, and social isolation was attributed to neglectful families. Commenters also suggested that alleviating social isolation was the responsibility of neighbours and volunteers. These three arguments accounted for 88% of the comments. Much less commonly, social isolation was described as due to the march of Western civilisation. This analysis shows how the public are active in their response to, and largely rejection of, framing social isolation as a public health issue. Although the health impacts of social isolation were endorsed, this was insufficient for structural explanations to prevail. Public health campaigners need to understand how individualising accounts of health issues are used to undermine public health explanations so as to most effectively challenge them.

Social isolation among older people has profound implications for health (Coyle & Dugan, 2012; Hawton, Green, & Dickens, 2011; Luanaigh & Lawlor, 2008). Social isolation refers to having a restricted social network and limited social contact (Holt-Lunstad, Smith, Baker, Harris, & Stephenson, 2015). Loneliness, the subjective experience of inadequate social contact, is also a cause and consequence of poor health. It is reported that loneliness will reach 'epidemic proportions' in the coming decade (Holt-Lunstad et al., 2015). A number of explanations have been provided for the increase in social isolation among older people, including increased geographical distance between family members, reduction in family size and social network size (Nicholson, 2012), and lack of transport and facilities to support social integration among older people.

The concern with loneliness and social isolation among older people has been reported in the media as a health concern as health damaging as smoking and obesity (Holt-Lunstad, Smith, & Layton, 2010; Holt-Lunstad et al., 2015). Social isolation is believed to be preventable and amenable to interventions at the community and population level (Wright-St Clair, Neville, Forsyth, White, & Napier, 2017). Understanding social isolation in terms of prevalence, drivers and outcomes supports the framing of social isolation as a public health concern. This is used to justify social isolation as a public issue, as a cost to society and as deserving of attention and remediation. However, there has been little analysis of how the public respond to media framing of social isolation as a public health issue.

The way social issues are framed by the media powerfully shapes public discourse and policy debates (Korn, Gibbins, & Azmier, 2003; Weathers & Kendall, 2015). Media frames influence the way people interpret issues, including the nature and causes of the problem, where responsibility lies, and potential solutions to address the problem (Jenkins, Signal, & Thomson, 2011; Kitzinger, 2007). The frame can be identified through signature rhetorical devices relating to the author's position (how they describe the issue and what they emphasise), suggested causal roots (what is identified as the main cause and where blame is laid), solutions proposed (who is responsible, what is included and excluded) and expressed core values (what values are evident) (Jenkins et al., 2011). As such, the framing of an issue by the media is a form of political influence, which promotes a particular interpretation through the selection, emphasis or omission or certain views, and can overlay moral judgements (Jenkins et al., 2011).

Audiences are not passive recipients of what they see and read in the media (Livingstone, 2004, 2005). Examining the response to media messages demonstrates how consumers are active in evaluating and resisting media content (Seale, 2003). The media also reflect public understandings; journalists shape the frames they use in terms of the anticipated views of their consumers in order to encourage repeated consumption of particular media outlets. In this way, the media shape how issues are framed whilst at the same time reflecting audience expectations for how social issues should be cast. Online discussion of news media provides a valuable site for examining audience response to media framing. Whilst there have long been interactive spaces for mediated public deliberations, such as talkback radio, the Internet offers more accessible, immediate and interactive forums. This opens up a democratic interactional space that allows large numbers of people to voice their opinions to wide audiences, an opportunity historically reserved for journalists (Hurley, Breheny, & Tuffin, 2017). Respondents are able to deliberate, draft and change their responses multiple times (Abele, 2011). The relative immediacy and anonymity of online interaction create an environment where people are more likely to contribute in uninhibited ways (Jowett, 2015). Although the journalistic content of online media is similar to print, commenting facilities on such articles provide an opportunity to consider both the media framing and the audience response to such frames (Kitzinger, 2004).

One in 10 elderly Kiwis could be 'socially isolated'

To show the negotiations between media portrayal and audience response, we chose a case study approach to one online article: 'One in 10 elderly Kiwis could be "socially isolated", Age Concern says' (Spink, 2016). This provided a way to examine how the media frame a social or health issue, and how readers take up, resist or reshape the frame provided (Kitzinger, 2004) in unsolicited naturalistic data. The article provided a useful case study as there was a substantial corpus of data and detailed commenting rather than surface agreement. The commenters responded both to the claims made in the article and to the comments posted by others. We examined this article and the comments to answer the following questions: What sort of problem is social isolation? Who is responsible for it? And what might the solutions be?

Method

Framing analysis draws attention to the frames that are used to shape a problem and asks: 'How is reality represented? How are key participants portrayed? How is the problem defined? Who is assigned responsibility for this issue? What solutions are presented' (Kitzinger, 2007, p. 157). Rhetorical analysis examines people in interaction to understand common sense ways of understanding and debating issues (Billig, 1991). The key feature of rhetorical analysis is argument. People engage in argument by expressing opinions, taking stances and through countering others' argumentative positions, either explicit or anticipated. This analysis uses framing analysis to identify how the problem of social isolation is defined and solutions advanced and rhetorical analysis to acknowledge the interactive nature of the data which includes argument and counter argument. As Kitzinger (2007) describes, words have powerful cultural resonance. Because of this, the whole frame need not be elaborated every time it is used; a condensed metaphor or trope can signify the frame an account is located within. The reader brings this shared understanding to contextualise short explanations, such as those provided in the comments.

Analytic method

The article 'One in 10 elderly Kiwis could be "socially isolated", Age Concern says' (Spink, 2016) generated 379 comments from readers of the online version of the article. This article was published on the highly accessed news site stuff.co.nz. This site is a subsidiary of Fairfax Media and boasts that it is 'New Zealand's #1 news site' with an audience of 1,905,000. Its readership is spread evenly across the adult age groups (Fairfax Media, 2016). This is an online news source in the public domain, and commenters expect that their comments will be viewed and evaluated without restriction. The original wording, spelling and punctuation in the comments have been reproduced in the extracts, and the user names are those provided by the commenters.

First, the article was analysed to understand how social isolation was framed. This involved close reading of the text alongside analysis of the embedded video content and photographs and captions. Following this, the comments were read and re-read to understand the overall claims being made about the source of and responsibility for social isolation among older people. At the end of this process, four overarching lines of argument, or frames, were identified that accounted for social isolation among older people: individuals, families, communities, and wider social changes. Once these predominant lines of reasoning were identified, the comments were systematically coded in terms of these accounts. Most of the comments fit simply into one code accounting for social isolation. Examples that best represented each of the ways of framing social isolation were used to illustrate the analysis and to demonstrate the implications of each frame for answering the questions posed above: How are people portrayed and the problem defined? Who is responsible? What solutions are possible? (Kitzinger, 2007).

Results

Dangerous as smoking 15 cigarettes a day

The headline of the article framed social isolation among older people at the outset in terms of prevalence: 'One in 10 elderly Kiwis could be "socially isolated"', signalling the public health framing used to represent the issue. Following this, the article personalised the issues of social isolation by foregrounding the situation of one particular older woman: 'There are days Lorna Batchelor gets so lonely she breaks down.' Through the text of the article, the embedded video and the photograph, this particular socially isolated older woman is illustrated as the face of a problem of social disintegration 'I've sat and broke down into tears sometimes. I say to myself, "Nobody cares. What am I doing here?"' This representation of the issue as located with one socially isolated older person reflects a standard media technique to personify the issue. The focus on Lorna links her experience with the experience of many other older people; the account becomes newsworthy because it reflects a common experience (Seale, 2003). This is strengthened with an embedded video of Lorna recounting Christmas Day spent alone. This video runs for just short of one and a half minutes and shows Lorna sitting alone in her living room. The living room is stereotypically that of an older person, containing crochet rugs on the chairs, older style furniture and dated décor. Lorna is conservatively dressed, grey haired and bespectacled. Close to tears, she narrates her desperation by claiming, 'I might as well be dead'. The video pans to show a clock's second hand ticking to suggest the slow passing of time. Cutting across this, Lorna introduces the notion that her family have their own lives, and that their happiness should be sufficient for her: 'As long as they're happy, it's great'.

Moving on from this personification of social isolation, the article directs the lens outward, by first linking Lorna's plight to the plight of other older people in the district of Canterbury (particularly poignant given the ongoing effects of the destructive Canterbury earthquakes of 2010/2011). 'Batchelor is one of an estimated 7000 elderly people in Christchurch living day-to-day with little to no interaction with the outside world.' This links loneliness to features of place and networks of services, strengthening the public health frame. The lens then shifts to social isolation as a national issue: 'Elderly advocates say social isolation among the nation's older population needs to be recognised as a serious issue'. This culminates in the framing of the destructive potential of social isolation as a public health problem: 'It's as dangerous to your health as smoking 15 cigarettes a day. We are social beings and we know we need social connection to maintain mentally and physically well'. Once the public health framing has been established, the article returns to focus on the character of this story, the lonely widow profiled at the beginning, represented in the video and pictured in the accompanying photograph. Her social isolation is linked to the growth of loneliness among older people to justify the expansion of services to address this need. The responding commentary can be understood in the light of this framing of social isolation as a personal tragedy linked to reduction in community services and the increasing alienation of older people from their communities.

Accounting for social isolation

The article framed social isolation as a public health issue with a tragic personal face. In response, the commenters did not trivialise or reject the health impacts of loneliness and social isolation. The comments supported the importance of social contact in maintaining health and well-being, not just in older age but for people of all ages. *PoppyT* linked loneliness to poor mental health and suicide: 'From experience – loneliness can lead to mental health issues, low self-esteem, and dare I say it, the will to end the suffering. I've been there and I am not afraid to admit it'. In this way, both the article and the comments linked social isolation to poor mental and physical health and used this to justify the importance of social integration. Instead of rejecting or trivialising social isolation, the comments focused on framing responsibility for social isolation. Most comments implicitly or explicitly answered the question posed by the poster *Cheshire cat*:

> So whose responsibility is it to provided social interaction for Lorna – is it her children's responsibility? Is it the state who should provide for that basic need? Should it fall to her neighbors because they happen to live in the house next door? Or should it fall upon Lorna?

Cheshire cat's rhetorical question covered the range of accounts provided to explain social isolation; responsibility is variously attributed to the lonely individual, the family, particular community members or the community as a whole, or the state.

Most of the comments were easily categorised in terms of one of these four predominant frames. Thirty-nine per cent of the comments situated social isolation as an individual problem. Older people were exhorted to join community groups, be kind to others or chastised for being unpleasant towards family and friends. Thirty per cent of the comments framed family as responsible for social isolation in later life. This was the case even if family members had not been devoted parents or grandparents. Nineteen per cent framed social isolation among older people as a community responsibility. The main thrust of this framing was that neighbours or volunteers should provide opportunities for socialising older people. Four per cent of the comments attributed social isolation to wider social change or globalisation. Nearly three per cent of the comments combined frames or located one frame within another, for example claiming that neglectful families were due to wider social changes. The remaining 5% could not be coded, often because they made statements of agreement without it being clear what they were agreeing to, corrected the spelling or punctuation of others, or introduced material unrelated to the topic.

Individual responsibility

The most common way of accounting for social isolation was to place responsibility squarely with each individual older person. Older people were urged to engage in a range of activities, enlist the services of others, or failing other alternatives, and take a positive attitude towards their situation. Individual responsibility extended to exhortations that older people should ensure they were pleasant to be around, treat their family members nicely over the life course, and maintain social connections proactively. These explanations ranged from gently phrased suggestions to sharply worded accusations like *red*'s response to the suggestion that more services are required: 'Nonsense. All the resources and in place and the care and people are too foolish to find their way'. Socially isolated people were viewed as having the freedom to make individual choices to alleviate isolation. This is best illustrated by commenter *justjoy*. In response to claims that Lorna has been badly treated, *justjoy* responds: 'She is not being treated like anything. Her kids have their own lives. They are not responsible for her happiness – we each make our own happiness and build our own futures'.

If they can, why can't this woman?
Individual responsibility for one's own future was developed into specific prescriptions for how people could best avoid social isolation in older age. Although acknowledging that there are individual circumstances such as mobility restrictions and limited access to transport, *oldlady* claims that the key lack is in older people not taking responsibility and concludes with, 'What's to stop Lorna doing that?' By finishing with this rhetorical question, *oldlady* dismisses the acknowledged issues of health and transport and instead focuses the argument on what Lorna could do to overcome these constraints. *LisaY* similarly balances her accounting of what causes social isolation, including health issues, with suggestions for overcoming these issues straight from individual health promotion advice:

> There are many reasons people become isolated – no matter what age. It could be depression, lack of mobility, or even over reliance on others to entertain. There many ways you can counteract this – even as simple as a beginning the day with a short walk.

Although acknowledging that each person has individual challenges to navigate, these challenges are not sufficient to override individual responsibility. Instead, they were an opportunity to hammer home the message that anything is possible, and older people need to 'at least give it a try' (*embeez452*). *Veruca* makes a similar claim, concluding: 'You CAN be happy – it's in your mind and you are in charge of that'.

Socially isolated older people are viewed as having the capacity to overcome their circumstances, if they made the right choices and had the right priorities. The main message from commenters is that older people cannot be passive, but must be proactive in their efforts to prevent and overcome loneliness: 'It is not everyone else's responsibility to babysit and make sure she is content with her day. It hers' (*Lydia Deetz*). In this way, health outcomes are a reward for 'good' behaviour, 'bad' behaviour is punished by social isolation and loneliness – and responsibility sits squarely with the older people themselves.

You reap what you sow
Another strong accounting for social isolation and loneliness as an individual responsibility was the notion that older people 'reap what they sow'. Loneliness in older age was viewed as a just consequence for poor social relationships in earlier life: 'I can't help but think "you reap what you sow". Loving families do care for one another and support one another' (*justjoy*). Similarly, the lack of involvement of her children in her life was used as evidence for her previous poor decisions and priorities: '0 out of 6 children. Wonder what her priorities as a mother were to them as kids' (*HalfAClue*). In recognition that an alternative frame exists that situates family as responsible for the social lives of their members, other commenters refuted this by saying that older people were individually responsible for how their families treated them, as this depended on how they had treated others earlier in life. 'No it is not the responsibility of her children. If she wanted their company in her old age, she shouldn't have made them so disillusioned with her that they chose to estrange themselves' (*Rosalain*).

Family obligations were viewed as a reflection of the individual behaviour of family members over time rather than in terms of a web of obligations to others. In this way, family relationships were constructed as freely chosen and dependent on meeting the expectations of others.

Shameful families

The second explanation framed social isolation as a family responsibility. This was epitomised by *CPR's* comment: 'I'm sorry, but where the hell is her family? Four out of her six children live in Canterbury and she has to spend Christmas day alone? They should be ashamed of themselves'. In the more uncompromising version of this frame, older people regardless of their conduct in earlier life are the ongoing responsibility of their immediate family. At times, a softer version of family responsibility was provided, which acknowledged that in rare cases the family members could have profoundly undermined their relationships to such a degree that family responsibility was fraught. Even in this situation, however, family members were exhorted to see beyond these situations and take responsibility for older family members: 'But there is a place for letting go and moving on' (*George63*). Taking responsibility in such cases was viewed as modelling appropriate caring relationships to their own children. Be mindful that your children can and often do learn from you so if you treat your parent badly, and 'judge them as a parent, you may well be teaching your children to treat you like that too' (*Cleo Selene*).

This account acknowledges the difficulties of many family situations but locates the responsibility for overcoming this in enduring family connections. In this account, family relationships are permanent and cannot be chosen based upon an evaluation of the conduct of the parents over the life course.

Neighbourly responsibility

This account suggests that all members of the community are responsible for alleviating loneliness. Generally, this involved calls for increased volunteering and formal services, but also included calls to know one's neighbours. Many of the commenters responded with a wish to alleviate this tragic representation of social isolation by volunteering for services to support older people, as *Mrs McC's* comment typifies:

> I would love to be able to help someone like this. Isn't there some kind of register, or did there used to be, where you could 'buddy' with someone like this and call them once or twice a week? Or something, anything?

Others pointed to existing services that provide a point of social contact for isolated older people. The need for people to generally be more supportive and welcoming was also mentioned by several commenters such as *Jan Kinloch* 'But I believe we as a society can change this epidemic of loneliness in our elderly. If we ALL reach out and take time to be friends to those lonely people live close to us, surely things can change!' *Rachel57* explicitly addressed the relative responsibility of children compared to the community to provide for its members in this way: 'How about a community where people care about their neighbours? This article raised an issue of loneliness when surrounded by people. Let's address that issue instead of blaming others and avoiding our own responsibility'. Although this frame pointed to the role of neighbours, community members or formal services, this remains an individual response 'our own responsibility', not requiring social or systemic change. In doing so, this framing suggested that responsibility for the social isolation of community members belonged to individual community members.

Western culture

This frame provided the most systemic account of the responsibility for social isolation. It was based on the notion that political goals, global change or the advance of Western civilisation has rightly or wrongly meant that older people have been abandoned. As *MrFloyd* illustrates:

> Our modern economic-based society is to blame.. The elderly don't contribute therefore don't matter... We have institutions to teach our young, where as in third world countries it is the elderlys job to pass on knowledge to the next generation, giving them a great sense of purpose and belonging.

Although *MrFloyd* and others bemoaned this state of affairs, it was often viewed as inevitable and as reflecting progress understood broadly. *Roslain* claims, 'In modern society, the younger generations often have far greater knowledge than the elderly, and also have numerous other more reliable sources of information if they need it'. Other commenters attributed social isolation to Western culture, but instead viewed this change as negative rather than progress: 'we are loosing out communities because we are all selfish. including the elderly. western culture at its best.' (*binthinkin*). Here, Western cultural change is reduced to individual personality defects such as selfishness.

At times, these accounts pointed to older people as collateral damage in political decision-making designed to reduce public spending. As *RonChad* describes:

> Most [commenters] seem to forget that the aim of health and social organisations has been, and still is, to keep the elderly in their own homes as long as possible. To bundle most elderly into residential care, with Govt., subsidies would destroy poor Bill English's [NZ Minister of Finance] surplus completely!

Commenters here acknowledge social context as a source of the problem and note social disintegration as a key factor, but the remedy is often still family members. As *speights56* describes here:

> The curse of western civilization, where the elderly are cast off by their families to live their lives out often in total isolation or nursing homes because they are to much trouble and yet in lands not far away the elder are treated respectfully and live within the family group.

Social and economic conditions are provided as an explanation, but the solution to social isolation is typically still the family group. Whilst focusing on the changing world, even these commenters propose solutions based on individual behaviour change, whether the individual is the person experiencing social isolation, their family member or neighbour.

Discussion

The online article framed social isolation as a public health problem. This framing was met with a strongly articulated response which located loneliness as a private trouble that reflected a lack of personal effort to avoid loneliness or a shameful family response. In this way, commenters blamed and shamed people for being lonely in later life and extended this shame to families that include lonely people (see McCartney, 2015). By urging individuals and their families to make better choices, these comments obscure material and societal conditions that shape social isolation. Some commenters placed the choices and behaviour of individuals within an environmental frame – social isolation as a symptom of wider social environments. These wider accounts noted changes in society and declining social relationships. However, the broader context of community environments and geographical contexts were not understood as the solution to social isolation. Lawrence (2004) describes the framing of social issues in the public domain as being on a continuum from individualising to systemic frames. The balance has shifted markedly towards an increasingly individualistic approach which foregrounds personal responsibility for health (Lawrence, 2004). In this case study, the majority of accounts reduce society to individuals, families and neighbours; individuals and families are exhorted to look to themselves, and wider social and community responsibility limited to neighbourliness. These individualising frames shift away from systemic and structural accounts of social isolation that might call for sustained social change.

Similarly, C Wright Mills' distinction between personal troubles and public issues is applicable here (Mills, 1959, 1967). Within the personal trouble frame, health is a personal responsibility; people are encouraged to make healthy choices and engage in healthy behaviour. In contrast, public issues are 'matters that transcend these local environments of the individual and the limited range of his life' (Mills, 1967, p. 396). The 'crisis of loneliness' as a personal trouble looks to the character of the individual, their skills and efforts. It is the fault of the individual if they are lonely. This framing creates distance from wider social determinants, such as the challenges of an ageing population, socioeconomic factors, and social and community structures. Individual control over social isolation is emphasised, and this prompts moralising judgements of isolated older people. This aligns with neoliberal principles of reducing government intervention, enhancing individual responsibility for outcomes and understanding inequality in outcomes as an inevitable consequence of poor individual choices (Ayo, 2012).

This analysis examined how commenters respond to the public health framing of social isolation. Those who post comments may not represent the range of views on the topic; people who largely disagree with the article framing may be more likely to respond. Online commenting provides space for voices of dissent, and so the prevalence of views may not reflect wider population views. What this analysis does provide is examination of the ways that within the highly social topic of social isolation, responsibility is mostly devolved to the individual and their family and neighbours. This demonstrates the difficulty that people have conceptualising issues as reflecting social and systemic causes.

Resisting an individualising frame

In this example, a complex social problem is framed as a public health concern; however, the comments largely resist this framing. The commenters argue that social resources should not be spent on alleviating private troubles. Locating social isolation as a private trouble avoids politicisation of isolation, minimising the need for political solutions (Baum, 2008). A public health frame explores the drivers and determinants of social isolation, the context, how it affects both individuals and populations, and identifies points for intervention, including opportunities to reduce inequalities between groups. As a public health issue, social isolation among older people can be viewed as an outcome of structural or political arrangements. Resistance to structural accounts of health issues may have implications for the level of support for public health interventions and policies. Investment in transport, services, urban planning and resourcing requires widespread public support. Without such support, public health advocacy may be undermined by arguments that locate responsibility not with communities, societies and governments but with individuals, families and neighbours.

There is space for the media to contribute to these broader understandings, to create a more favourable environment for public health action to tackle social isolation. However, public health advocates need to engage with the resistance people may have to such accounts of social isolation. The shift from welfare liberalism to a neoliberal position significantly shapes the focus and policy of public health and health promotion through the reduction of government intervention, increased privatisation and promotion of the ethos that people are self-regulating individuals (Baum & Fisher, 2014). To challenge these individual understandings, public health advocates may need to engage with both media representation and response to convincingly reframe health risk as located with the wider environment which structures possibilities for all people (Lawrence, 2004).

The audience for public health messages are active negotiators of the material they are presented (Livingstone, 2013). Livingstone (2004) discusses the distinction between the audience and the public. The audience are often viewed as passive private individuals receiving a delivered message (Livingstone, 2004). In contrast, the public tend to be viewed as active and engaged citizens. This distinction may provide insight into this analysis. The online article hailed an audience with a message regarding the cause of social isolation among older people. By commenting on the article, members of this audience demonstrate that they are not passive recipients of this message, but active participants in public health debate.

Recognising this active negotiation and using it to shape the debate may encourage engagement with a public health frame in the media. As Seale (2003) notes, media accounts are often convincing because they use familiar turns of phrase to encourage audiences to respond in predictable ways. Words have powerful cultural significance, and particular metaphors or tropes signify broader conceptual frames (Kitzinger, 2007). In this analysis, the success of some people is used to chastise others for their failure: 'if they can, why can't this woman?' and to suggest that outcomes in life are fairly distributed according to life conduct 'you reap what you sow'. Such turns of phrase signify an individualising frame of personal responsibility for outcomes. However, such phrases could be strategically employed to trouble these individualising frames. Rhetorically, these turns of phrase could be used to compare societies as well as used to chastise people for individual outcomes. 'If they can, why can't others' could equally be used to account for the distribution of opportunities between societies: if social arrangements in one context can produce equitable outcomes, then these outcomes should be able to be replicated elsewhere. Similarly, if individuals reap what they sow, then equally societies reap what they sow: a foundation of social justice will reap equality of outcomes at a societal level. Rather than avoiding these turns of phrase because they are identifiable as belonging to an individualising argument, the logic they use can be re-purposed to point to the societal reproduction of opportunities and outcomes. Reframing individualising rhetorical devices in terms of structural accounts may be a powerful tool for bringing about public health change.

Social isolation among older people is shaped by social structures and dominant discourses. Attributing social isolation to poor choices and family inadequacy needs to be challenged to improve the public health of older people. Challenging these accounts strategically and persuasively through the media is one way to achieve this. Using the language of personal responsibility for health to advocate structural change may be a more persuasive strategy to promote a public health framing of social isolation.

Disclosure statement

No potential conflict of interest was reported by the authors.

ORCID

Mary Breheny ⓘD http://orcid.org/0000-0002-1603-8033

References

Abele, S. (2011). Social interaction in cyberspace: Social construction with few constraints. In Z. Birchmeier, B. Dietz-Uhler, & G. Stasser (Eds.), *Strategic uses of social technology: An interactive perspective of social psychology* (pp. 84–107). New York, NY: Cambridge University Press.

Ayo, N. (2012). Understanding health promotion in a neoliberal climate and the making of health conscious citizens. *Critical Public Health, 22*(1), 99–105.

Baum, F. (2008). *The new public health* (3rd ed.). Melbourne: Oxford University Press.

Baum, F., & Fisher, M. (2014). Why behavioural health promotion endures despite its failure to reduce health inequities. *Sociology of Health & Illness, 36*(2), 213–225.

Billig, M. (1991). *Ideology and opinions: Studies in rhetorical psychology*. London: Sage.

Coyle, C. E., & Dugan, E. (2012). Social isolation, loneliness and health among older adults. *Journal of Aging and Health, 24*, 1346–1363.

Fairfax Media. (2016). Stuff media kit. Retrieved November 17, 2016, from http://static.stuff.co.nz/stuff/advertise-online/Media_Kit.pdf

Hawton, A., Green, C., & Dickens, A. P. (2011). The impact of social isolation on the health status and health-related quality of life of older people. *Quality of Life Research, 20*(1), 57–67.

Holt-Lunstad, J., Smith, T. B., & Layton, J. B. (2010). Social relationships and mortality risk: A meta-analytic review. *PLoS Med, 7*(7), e1000316.

Holt-Lunstad, J., Smith, T. B., Baker, M., Harris, T., & Stephenson, D. (2015). Loneliness and social isolation as risk factors for mortality: A meta-analytic review. *Perspectives on Psychological Science, 10*(2), 227–237.

Hurley, K., Breheny, M., & Tuffin, K. (2017). Intergenerational inequity arguments and the implications for state-funded financial support of older people. *Ageing & Society, 37*(3), 561–580.

Jenkins, C. L., Signal, L., & Thomson, G. (2011). Framing obesity: The framing contest between industry and public health at the New Zealand inquiry into obesity. *Obesity Reviews, 12*, 1022–1030.

Jowett, A. (2015). A case for using online discussion forums in critical psychological research. *Qualitative Research in Psychology, 12*(3), 287–297.

Kitzinger, J. (2004). Audience and readership research. In J. D. H. Downing, D. McQuail, P. Schlesinger, & E. Wartella (Eds.), *Sage handbook of media studies* (pp. 167–182). Thousand Oaks, CA: Sage.

Kitzinger, J. (2007). Framing and frame analysis. In E. Devereaux (Ed.), *Media studies: Key issues and debates* (pp. 134–161). London: Sage.

Korn, D., Gibbins, R., & Azmier, J. (2003). Framing public policy towards a public health paradigm for gambling. *Journal of Gambling Studies, 19*(2), 235–256.

Lawrence, R. G. (2004). Framing obesity: The evolution of news discourse on a public health issue. *Press/Politics, 9*(3), 56–75.

Livingstone, S. (2004). The challenge of changing audiences. Or, what is the audience researcher to do in the age of the internet? *European Journal of Communication, 19*(1), 75–86.

Livingstone, S. (2005). On the relation between audiences and publics. In S. Livingstone (Ed.), *Audiences and publics: When cultural engagement matters for the public sphere. Changing media – changing Europe series (2)* (pp. 17–41). Bristol: Intellect Books.

Livingstone, S. (2013). The participation paradigm in audience research. *The Communication Review, 16*(1–2), 21–30. doi: 10.1080/10714421.2013.757174

Luanaigh, C. Ó., & Lawlor, B.A. (2008). Loneliness and the health of older people. *International Journal of Geriatric Psychiatry, 23*, 1213–1221.

McCartney, M. (2015). The government's plan to blame and shame people for having disease. *BMJ, 351*, h4368. doi:10.1136/bmj.h4368

Mills, C. W. (1959). *The sociological imagination*. New York, NY: Oxford University Press.

Mills, C. W. (1967). *Power, politics and people. The collective essays of C. Wright Mills*. New York, NY: Oxford University Press.

Nicholson, N. R. (2012). A review of social isolation: An important but underassessed condition in older adults. *Journal of Primary Prevention, 33*, 137–152.

Seale, C. (2003). Health and media: An overview. *Sociology of Health & Illness, 25*(6), 513–531.

Spink, E. (2016). *One in 10 elderly Kiwis could be 'socially isolated', Age Concern says*. Retrieved from http://www.stuff.co.nz/national/health/76229784/One-in-10-elderly-Kiwis-could-be-socially-isolated-Age-Concern-says

Weathers, M. R., & Kendall, B. E. (2015). Developments in the framing of climate change as a public health issue in US newspapers. *Environmental Communication, 10*(5), 593–611. doi:10.1080/17524032.2015.1050436

Wright-St Clair, V. A., Neville, S., Forsyth, V., White, L., & Napier, S. (2017). Integrative review of older adult loneliness and social isolation in Aotearoa/New Zealand. *Australasian Journal of Ageing, 36*(2), 114–123. doi:10.1111/ajag.12379

Index